# Women Self-Improvement Book

CRAFTED BY SKRIUWER

**Copyright © 2024 by Skriuwer.**

All rights reserved. No part of this book may be used or reproduced in any form whatsoever without written permission except in the case of brief quotations in critical articles or reviews.

For more information, contact : **kontakt@skriuwer.com** (www.skriuwer.com)

# TABLE OF CONTENTS

## CHAPTER 1: DISCOVERING YOUR TRUE SELF AND GOALS

- *Exploring self-reflection to reveal your authentic path*
- *Learning how personal values shape meaningful life objectives*

## CHAPTER 2: BUILDING SELF-ESTEEM AND CONFIDENCE

- *Understanding self-worth and dismantling negative beliefs*
- *Using practical techniques to boost daily confidence*

## CHAPTER 3: HEALTHY HABITS FOR BODY AND MIND

- *Crafting a balanced lifestyle through nutrition and movement*
- *Staying mentally refreshed with simple, consistent self-care routines*

## CHAPTER 4: EMOTIONAL HEALING AND GROWTH

- *Addressing inner wounds and finding pathways to forgiveness*
- *Transforming pain into lessons for deeper personal understanding*

## CHAPTER 5: EFFECTIVE COMMUNICATION IN EVERYDAY LIFE

- *Listening actively to foster better relationships*
- *Speaking with clarity, respect, and empathy*

## CHAPTER 6: SETTING BOUNDARIES AND PROTECTING YOUR ENERGY

- Learning to say "no" without guilt to maintain emotional balance
- Establishing healthy limits in personal and professional settings

## CHAPTER 7: OVERCOMING FEAR AND ANXIETY

- Identifying triggers and adopting calming strategies
- Confronting worries step by step with courage and self-compassion

## CHAPTER 8: FINDING BALANCE AND MANAGING STRESS

- Prioritizing tasks and avoiding burnout through smart planning
- Using mindful breaks and simple techniques to reduce tension

## CHAPTER 9: PERSONAL VALUES AND LIFE PURPOSE

- Discovering guiding principles that anchor your decisions
- Aligning daily choices with your deeper sense of meaning

## CHAPTER 10: CAREER GROWTH AND PROFESSIONAL DEVELOPMENT

- Defining clear goals for advancement and skill-building
- Navigating workplace challenges with assertiveness and adaptability

## CHAPTER 11: NURTURING SUPPORTIVE RELATIONSHIPS

- *Recognizing healthy dynamics that uplift and encourage*
- *Strengthening trust, empathy, and conflict resolution skills*

---

## CHAPTER 12: SELF-CARE AND RELAXATION

- *Recharging physically and emotionally through daily rituals*
- *Creating personal routines that ease stress and promote calm*

---

## CHAPTER 13: BALANCING FAMILY, FRIENDS, AND PERSONAL SPACE

- *Protecting time for yourself while showing up for loved ones*
- *Avoiding burnout by honoring your own needs and boundaries*

---

## CHAPTER 14: CREATIVITY AND SELF-DISCOVERY

- *Tapping into artistic or innovative outlets for deeper insight*
- *Using curiosity and playful exploration to expand your horizons*

---

## CHAPTER 15: POSITIVE THINKING AND GROWTH MINDSET

- *Replacing limiting beliefs with empowering self-talk*
- *Viewing challenges as opportunities for learning and progress*

---

## CHAPTER 16: ADAPTING TO CHANGE AND LIFE CHALLENGES

- *Staying flexible and open-minded when routines shift*
- *Turning unexpected obstacles into stepping stones for growth*

## CHAPTER 17: LEADERSHIP AND INFLUENCE

- *Guiding and inspiring others with empathy and authenticity*
- *Practicing ethical persuasion and building trust in any setting*

---

## CHAPTER 18: FINANCIAL INDEPENDENCE AND RESPONSIBILITY

- *Mastering budgeting, saving, and mindful spending*
- *Developing long-term strategies for security and empowerment*

---

## CHAPTER 19: BUILDING EMOTIONAL RESILIENCE

- *Learning to bounce back from setbacks with self-compassion*
- *Adapting healthy outlets for processing difficult emotions*

---

## CHAPTER 20: SUSTAINING GROWTH AND NEXT STEPS

- *Reflecting on progress and setting new personal challenges*
- *Maintaining balance, curiosity, and purpose throughout life*

---

## EPILOGUE: LIVING YOUR GROWTH JOURNEY

- *Carrying forward the lessons and embracing continuous learning*
- *Trusting yourself as the ultimate source of ongoing transformation*

# Chapter 1: Discovering Your True Self and Goals

## Introduction

Every person has a unique set of thoughts, feelings, and dreams. Sometimes, though, we get stuck in routines that make us feel like we are living someone else's life. We may struggle to find what truly drives us, or we might ignore that small, persistent voice inside that calls us toward something bigger. This chapter is about helping you find your own path and purpose. It will guide you through the process of self-discovery and help you learn how to set goals that reflect your true self.

Discovering who you really are can be a scary thought at first. You might worry that you are not "good enough" or that the real you is too different from what other people expect. These fears are normal, but they should not stop you from becoming comfortable with your own identity. The aim here is to help you see that your uniqueness is an asset, not a problem. When you embrace who you are, you can set goals that inspire you and bring excitement to your life.

## Understanding Self-Discovery

Self-discovery is the process of learning about yourself on a deeper level. It includes understanding your emotions, your habits, and the reasons behind your daily actions. A lot of people walk through life without asking themselves why they do certain things. When you look closer, you often uncover interesting insights that can help you make better decisions.

Self-discovery also means recognizing the values you hold close. Values are the beliefs or ideas you consider important, such as honesty, kindness, adventure, stability, and so on. When you know your core values, you can shape your life around them. This makes it easier to see if something is aligned with who you are or if it goes against your natural flow.

### Why It's Important

- **Clarity**: When you understand yourself, you gain clarity about what you want. This clarity helps you avoid making random choices that do not serve you in the long run.
- **Confidence**: Knowing yourself also boosts self-confidence. You trust your instincts more and are less likely to be swayed by others' opinions.
- **Direction**: Self-discovery gives you a direction. Instead of wandering through life, you can move forward with a sense of purpose.

## Starting the Journey: Reflecting on Yourself

The first step in self-discovery is taking time to reflect. Reflection means thinking deeply about your thoughts, emotions, and experiences. One of the simplest ways to reflect is through journaling. You do not have to be a great writer or have fancy tools. All you need is a notebook (or a simple app on your phone) and some privacy. Write about your day, your worries, or your dreams. The more honest you are on the page, the better you will understand yourself.

You can also reflect by asking yourself questions:

1. **What activities make me feel happy or calm?**
2. **What are my biggest fears and why do I have them?**
3. **What kind of people do I admire, and what qualities do they have?**
4. **How do I react to stress and conflict, and what can I learn from my reactions?**
5. **What have I always wanted to try, but felt too scared or too busy to do?**

These questions can lead to surprising answers that reveal passions or worries you had not fully acknowledged. Make sure to be patient with yourself. Self-discovery is not something that happens overnight.

## Observing Your Feelings Without Judgment

Many women struggle with negative self-talk or guilt when they try to explore their true selves. You might look back at past decisions and feel embarrassed. Or you might feel pressure to act a certain way because of cultural or family expectations. It is important to observe these feelings without judging yourself too harshly. Recognize them, then let them pass.

## A Simple Exercise

Close your eyes and take several deep breaths. Pay attention to any thoughts that pop into your head. Observe them, but imagine they are passing clouds in the sky. You do not have to chase them or block them. Let them drift in and out of your mind. This practice can help you become aware of your thoughts without letting them control you. Over time, this approach will help you accept yourself more fully.

## Identifying Your Strengths and Weaknesses

An important part of self-discovery is acknowledging both what you do well and what you struggle with. Sometimes we focus too much on our weaknesses and forget our strengths. Other times, we ignore our weaknesses to avoid feeling vulnerable. True growth happens when you know both sides and are willing to learn from them.

- **Strengths**: These can be talents, like being good at cooking, writing, or leading a team. They can also be personality traits, such as being empathetic, patient, or energetic.
- **Weaknesses**: These are areas where you may need more practice or better tools. For instance, you might be disorganized, easily stressed, or overly shy. It is okay to admit these areas and to seek ways to improve them.

By listing your strengths and weaknesses, you can see more clearly what might help you reach your goals and what may hold you back. You do not have to "fix" all your weaknesses at once, or even at all. Some weaknesses might not affect the life path you desire. However, being aware of them prevents surprises and helps you plan better.

## Discovering Your Core Values

Your values are personal beliefs that matter most to you. They guide your actions and help shape your sense of self. Sometimes, people do not even realize what their core values are until they have to make a tough decision.

Here is a short process to identify your values:

1. Think of moments in your life when you felt most fulfilled. What was happening then? How did you behave?
2. Write down any principles or ideas that come to mind, like honesty, family, freedom, creativity, or growth.
3. Narrow this list to five or six values. Pick the ones that truly light a spark in you.
4. Reflect on how your current life matches or clashes with these values.

When you live in harmony with your values, you feel more at peace. If something you do contradicts your values, you are likely to experience discomfort. Discovering your values is key to living an authentic life.

## Setting Goals Based on Who You Are

Goals are often discussed as if they are something you just pick at random: lose weight, earn a certain amount of money, or get a new job. But meaningful goals should connect to your true self. If you set goals that go against your values, you will likely feel unmotivated or unhappy.

### Short-Term vs. Long-Term Goals

- **Short-Term Goals**: These can be small changes or tasks you want to achieve soon. For instance, you might aim to eat home-cooked meals at least three times a week, or read a new book each month. They give you quick wins and keep you energized.
- **Long-Term Goals**: These are bigger aspirations that require more time and planning. Examples include learning a new skill for a career change, saving for a house, or building a strong network of friends in a new city.

Balancing both short-term and long-term goals ensures that you have small steps to take now, while still aiming for bigger objectives in the future.

## The Role of Passion and Curiosity

Passion fuels our drive to explore, create, or excel. Some of us know exactly what we are passionate about, while others need time to discover it. If you are unsure, ask yourself what topics or activities grab your attention so much that you lose track of time. That is often a sign of passion.

Curiosity is related to passion but is more about being open-minded. Even if you do not feel a strong passion yet, try to stay curious. Read books about new subjects, talk to people from different walks of life, and attend events you usually would avoid. Curiosity leads to discovery, which can bloom into a passion over time.

## Embracing Your Unique Path

Part of self-discovery is accepting that your path is your own. Society, friends, and family may have certain expectations. While their input can be useful, you must decide which direction to take. This is especially important for women, who might feel torn between traditional roles and personal ambitions. Remember, there is no one "right" path for everyone.

You might worry about making mistakes if you choose a path that feels uncertain. Mistakes, however, are a natural part of growth. They help you learn more about yourself and refine your choices. What matters is listening to your inner guide and allowing yourself room to experiment.

## Overcoming Common Obstacles

The road to self-discovery is not always smooth. Here are a few obstacles that may pop up:

1. **Fear of Judgment**: You might be afraid of what people will say if you pursue something new or share your honest feelings. Know that judgment often comes from people's own insecurities. Focus on what makes sense for you.
2. **Self-Doubt**: It is common to question your abilities. Self-doubt can stop you from trying at all. Remind yourself that nobody starts off perfect and that growth comes with practice.
3. **Overthinking**: Some of us get lost in too many "what-if" scenarios. While planning is good, too much thinking can lead to paralysis. Take small steps and see what happens.
4. **Time Constraints**: Between work, family, and daily chores, you might feel you have no time to reflect. Consider scheduling brief moments (even 10 minutes a day) for self-reflection or journaling.

By learning to navigate these obstacles, you give yourself permission to explore. Small efforts build up over time, and each new insight will bring you closer to your true self.

## A Gentle Reminder About Self-Compassion

On your journey, self-compassion is essential. You might discover parts of yourself you do not like. You might realize you have made decisions that do not fit your values. Instead of beating yourself up, think of it as a positive sign that you now see where changes are needed. Thank yourself for having the courage to face these truths. Then, plan how you can move forward with more alignment to your real self.

## Putting It All Together

Let's do a brief summary of what we have covered:

- **Self-discovery** involves understanding your feelings, habits, strengths, weaknesses, and values.
- **Reflection** (through journaling or deep thought) helps you notice patterns and learn from your experiences.
- **Identifying values** clarifies what is important to you. This, in turn, helps you shape your goals.
- **Setting goals** that match your authentic self increases motivation and fulfillment.

## A Final Word

Finding who you are is a rewarding experience that can open many doors. It provides you with a sense of direction and a roadmap for your goals. Always remember that this is a personal journey. You will grow and change over time, and that is perfectly normal. The important thing is to keep checking in with yourself, adjusting your goals, and staying true to your values along the way.

The next chapter will focus on **Building Self-Esteem and Confidence**, which goes hand in hand with understanding yourself. Once you have a clearer sense of who you are, you can begin to feel more certain in your choices. This shift in mindset will help you step forward with less fear and more excitement about what lies ahead.

# Chapter 2: Building Self-Esteem and Confidence

## Introduction

Self-esteem is how you view your own worth as a person. Confidence is your belief in your ability to handle tasks and challenges. When you have healthy self-esteem, you see that you deserve respect and kindness, no matter what mistakes you have made or what others think. Confidence, on the other hand, helps you take action and reach your goals. Both self-esteem and confidence are important for living a balanced, fulfilling life.

Women often face social pressures that can harm their self-esteem. Messages from media, cultural expectations, and even well-meaning friends or family can make you doubt your strengths and question whether you are good enough. This chapter aims to help you build a strong foundation of self-esteem and confidence, so you can move through life with courage and optimism.

## Understanding the Difference Between Self-Esteem and Confidence

It is helpful to understand how self-esteem and confidence differ but also how they work together.

- **Self-Esteem**: This is your overall sense of personal value. If you have high self-esteem, you believe you are worthy of love and respect. You recognize that you, like everyone else, have flaws, but those flaws do not make you less deserving of happiness.
- **Confidence**: This is about what you think you can do. People can be confident in specific skills, like painting or speaking in public, even if they sometimes have doubts in other areas of life.

When self-esteem and confidence are both strong, you feel comfortable trying new things because you trust yourself. Even when you fail at something, you do not see it as proof that you are "not good enough." Instead, you see it as a chance to learn and improve.

## Root Causes of Low Self-Esteem

Before you can improve your self-esteem, it helps to look at why it might be low in the first place. Some common causes include:

1. **Negative Childhood Experiences**: If you grew up hearing a lot of criticism, you might have learned to believe that there is something wrong with you.
2. **Traumatic Events**: Physical or emotional abuse can cause deep wounds that make it hard to feel worthwhile.
3. **Unrealistic Standards**: Society often sets impossible beauty or success standards, causing many women to feel they do not measure up.
4. **Comparing Yourself to Others**: Constantly measuring yourself against others can lead to feelings of inadequacy.

These root causes might not disappear overnight, but awareness is the first step toward healing. By knowing why your self-esteem might be low, you can take steps to correct harmful beliefs and start building yourself up again.

## Practical Ways to Improve Self-Esteem

Raising your self-esteem takes consistent effort, but it is doable. Here are some approaches:

1. **Positive Self-Talk**: Pay attention to how you speak to yourself in your mind. Replace harsh or self-critical words with gentler, supportive language. For example, change "I messed up, I'm so stupid" to "I made a mistake, but I can learn from this."
2. **Surround Yourself with Positivity**: The people around you can influence your self-esteem. Try to spend time with those who uplift you, and limit your interactions with those who constantly criticize or belittle you. This does not always mean you can avoid them completely, but you can choose how often you see them or how seriously you take their opinions.
3. **Celebrate Small Achievements**: Every step forward counts. If you cooked a new recipe, finished a difficult work project, or went for a walk instead of sitting on the couch, celebrate that. Acknowledging little victories can help you feel more capable.

4. **Engage in Self-Care**: Make time for activities that soothe and recharge you. This can be a warm bath, reading a book, or going for a walk in nature. When you treat yourself with kindness, you send your mind the message that you are worth caring for.
5. **Set Realistic Expectations**: If you aim for perfection all the time, you might always feel disappointed. Learn to set goals that are challenging yet achievable. That way, you can feel accomplished rather than defeated.

## Confidence-Building Techniques

Confidence is closely tied to self-esteem, but it often has more to do with action. If you want to feel more confident in a certain area, you have to practice. Here are some ideas:

1. **Skill Development**
   If you lack confidence in public speaking, for example, you can take a public speaking course or practice with friends. The same goes for other tasks: the more you develop your skills, the more you trust yourself to do well.
2. **Visualization**
   Sometimes called "mental rehearsal," this technique involves picturing yourself doing something successfully. If you have a job interview, close your eyes and see yourself walking in calmly, answering questions with clarity, and leaving with a smile. This method can lower anxiety and boost performance.
3. **Start Small**
   If you try to do something far outside your comfort zone right away, you might become overwhelmed. Instead, take small steps. For example, if you want to become more confident socially, practice speaking up in small groups before diving into large events.
4. **Track Your Progress**
   Keep a journal or checklist of the steps you take to build confidence. Seeing how far you have come can inspire you to keep going, even when you face setbacks.

## Changing Limiting Beliefs

Limiting beliefs are ideas you hold about yourself that keep you from reaching your full potential. They often start with thoughts like "I can't do this," "I'm not smart enough," or "I don't deserve good things." Over time, these beliefs can become so ingrained that you no longer question them.

### How to Challenge Limiting Beliefs

- **Recognize Them**: Notice when these beliefs show up. For instance, if you think "I'll never be able to learn this skill," pause and recognize that thought as a belief, not a fact.
- **Question Them**: Ask yourself, "Is this always true?" or "Is there any proof that I can't do this?" Often, you will find evidence that you can learn if you try.
- **Replace Them**: Create new, more supportive beliefs like "I'm capable of learning new things" or "I am strong enough to handle challenges." Each time the old belief pops up, remind yourself of the new one.

This process takes time, but every effort brings you closer to a mindset that supports your growth instead of holding you back.

## The Role of Body Language

How you carry your body can affect how you feel about yourself. Standing up straight, making eye contact, and speaking clearly can increase your sense of confidence. Even if you are feeling unsure, adopting confident body language can help shift your mindset.

For example, if you tend to hunch your shoulders or look down, practice standing tall with your shoulders back and your chin up. At first, it might feel awkward, but over time, your posture can positively affect your mood and energy level.

## Avoiding Overconfidence and Arrogance

While confidence is a positive quality, it can sometimes slip into arrogance. Arrogance is the belief that you are better than others. This attitude can push people away and block your personal growth because you stop listening to feedback. True confidence includes humility and the ability to recognize when you have more to learn.

If you find yourself dismissing others' ideas or feeling superior, take a moment to ask why. Is there an insecurity beneath that feeling? Do you worry that someone else's success might overshadow your own? By being aware of such thoughts, you can keep your confidence grounded in respect for yourself and others.

## Building a Supportive Environment

When you are trying to improve your self-esteem and confidence, having a supportive environment makes a difference. This can include:

- **Friends Who Cheer You On**: Seek out friendships where both parties encourage each other's growth.
- **Mentors and Role Models**: Look for people who are already doing what you aspire to do. They can offer advice, guidance, and inspiration.
- **Positive Media**: The images, books, and videos you consume can affect your mindset. Choose sources that uplift you rather than tear you down.

## Dealing with Setbacks

No matter how hard you work on yourself, you will face setbacks. These might be job rejections, relationship problems, or simply a bad day where you doubt yourself. The important thing is how you respond to these setbacks.

1. **Accept the Situation**: It is okay to feel disappointed or sad. Let yourself feel those emotions without shame.
2. **Look for Lessons**: After you have calmed down, think about what you can learn. Maybe you gained a new perspective or discovered a weak spot you can improve.
3. **Move Forward**: Take the lesson and keep going. Remind yourself that setbacks are part of life, not signs of your inability.

## Affirmations and Encouragement

Affirmations are positive statements you say to yourself to challenge negative thoughts. Examples could be "I am strong," "I can handle what life brings," or "I love and respect myself." While they might feel cheesy at first, repeating affirmations can help shift your inner dialogue over time.

If you are comfortable, say them out loud in front of a mirror. Seeing your own face while speaking kindly to yourself can create a powerful emotional impact. Even if you do not fully believe the words at first, keep going. Over time, your mind starts to accept these messages.

## Balancing Self-Esteem with Self-Awareness

As you build your self-esteem, you also want to remain aware of your behavior and how it affects those around you. High self-esteem does not mean ignoring other people's feelings or shutting out criticism. In fact, having a healthy sense of self-worth often makes you more open to feedback, because you are not as threatened by it.

When you are honest about both your strengths and your weaknesses, you stay grounded. You can be proud of what you do well while still working on areas where you need growth. This balance allows you to keep growing without being too hard on yourself.

## Sustaining Your Growth

Building self-esteem and confidence is not a one-time event. It is a lifelong process. You may reach a point where you feel comfortable in your own skin, only to find that a major life change (like a new job, moving to a new city, or a big family event) shakes your confidence. That is normal.

Keep the following points in mind to sustain your growth:

- **Regular Self-Check-Ins**: Spend a few minutes each day or week reviewing your thoughts and progress. Ask yourself if any negative patterns are sneaking back in.
- **Ongoing Learning**: Take new courses, read books, or seek mentors who can help you grow. Expanding your skills and knowledge boosts confidence.
- **Healthy Boundaries**: Learn to say no when you need to. Protecting your time and energy supports both self-esteem and confidence. (Boundaries will be addressed in depth in a later chapter, so we will not repeat it here.)

# Chapter 3: Healthy Habits for Body and Mind

## Introduction

Caring for your body and mind helps set a strong foundation for everything else in life. When you feel healthy and energized, you can better handle challenges, build confidence, and stay focused on your goals. But health is not just about hitting the gym or following a strict diet. It includes the small daily decisions that shape how you think, feel, and act.

In this chapter, we will discuss ways to look after yourself physically and mentally. You will learn practical tips on nutrition, movement, rest, and mental well-being. These suggestions are not meant to be medical advice—always check with a healthcare professional before starting a new exercise or diet plan. Think of these ideas as tools to help you find what works best for you.

## The Mind-Body Connection

Your mind and body communicate constantly. When you are stressed or worried, you might feel a headache or tight muscles in your shoulders. On the flip side, when your body is healthy—well-fed, rested, and active—your mind often feels clearer and calmer. This link goes both ways, which means taking care of one side helps the other. By adopting healthy routines for your body, you set up conditions for a healthier mind. And by managing your thoughts, you can reduce stress, which benefits your body.

## Balanced Nutrition

One key to feeling your best is eating in a way that nourishes your body with the right balance of nutrients. Instead of thinking about strict diets or punishing yourself, try to focus on variety and balance.

1. **Whole Foods First**: Look for fresh vegetables, fruits, grains, and proteins. This means trying to limit overly processed foods that come in packages with lots of additives and sugar.

2. **Listen to Your Hunger and Fullness**: Your body often gives signals about when it is hungry or satisfied. Pay attention to these signs instead of forcing yourself to eat or skip meals based on the clock alone.
3. **Stay Hydrated**: Drinking enough water helps with digestion, mood, and energy levels. If you find plain water boring, you can add slices of lemon, cucumber, or fresh mint for flavor.
4. **Moderation, Not Perfection**: You do not have to cut out favorite treats. It is more about enjoying them in moderation. Life should include pleasure, and food can be part of that.

Balanced eating can also boost your immune system and protect you from certain illnesses in the long run. If you have specific questions or concerns about your diet, consult a registered dietitian or doctor who can guide you. The main point is to create a relationship with food that nourishes you without guilt or extremes.

## Movement and Exercise

Movement keeps your muscles strong, your heart healthy, and your mind more relaxed. Exercise also releases chemicals in your brain (like endorphins) that can lower stress and improve mood. But "exercise" does not always mean going to the gym every day. Here are some simple ways to stay active:

- **Walking**: Take a brisk walk around your neighborhood or local park. Even short walks can add up to big benefits over time.
- **Dancing**: Put on music you enjoy and dance in your living room. This not only burns calories but can also boost your mood.
- **Bodyweight Exercises**: Simple moves like squats, lunges, and push-ups can be done at home without equipment.
- **Stretching or Yoga**: Light stretching or basic yoga poses can improve flexibility and reduce muscle tension. If you can, look for beginner-friendly yoga videos or classes.

Try different types of movement to see what feels good. Some people love running; others prefer swimming or biking. The key is finding something that you enjoy so you are more likely to stick with it. Aim for consistency rather than perfection. Even a little physical activity each day can make a difference.

## Quality Sleep

Sleep is often overlooked, but it is essential for overall health. During sleep, your body and brain repair themselves. Lack of sleep can lead to poor focus, low energy, and even weight gain. Here are some tips for better sleep:

1. **Regular Sleep Schedule**: Try to go to bed and wake up at roughly the same time each day, even on weekends. This helps your body set an internal clock.
2. **Wind Down Before Bed**: Avoid bright screens and heavy meals close to bedtime. Instead, try a relaxing activity, like gentle reading or listening to calm music.
3. **Comfortable Environment**: Make your bedroom a peaceful place. Keep the temperature comfortable and the lights dim. Some people find that a small fan or sound machine helps create a soothing atmosphere.
4. **Limit Stimulants**: Caffeine and nicotine can disrupt your ability to fall asleep, especially if used later in the day. Be mindful of when and how much you consume.

A good night's sleep can greatly improve your mood, concentration, and overall well-being. If you struggle with chronic sleep problems, consider talking to a healthcare provider for specialized help.

## Mental Hygiene

Just like brushing your teeth, it is important to keep your mind clean and healthy. Mental hygiene refers to habits that keep your thoughts and emotions in a balanced state.

### Mindful Breaks

Taking short breaks throughout the day to pause, breathe, or quietly observe your surroundings can do wonders for your stress levels. Even a minute or two of deep breathing can reset a busy mind. If you work at a desk or spend hours taking care of family, schedule tiny moments to step away and let your mind rest.

**Limiting Mental Overload**

In our modern world, it is easy to get overwhelmed by a constant flow of information—news, social media, and more. Try to be mindful of how much information you consume. Set time limits on social media or use apps that remind you to take breaks. You do not have to read every comment or reply to every notification right away. Prioritize your mental health by allowing yourself time to unplug.

**Engaging Hobbies**

Hobbies are not just for fun; they can help you relax, increase creativity, and build a sense of achievement. Whether it is painting, playing an instrument, gardening, knitting, or learning a new language, hobbies help shift your focus away from stress. Pick something you like, and do not worry if you are not "good" at it at first. The main goal is to enjoy the process.

## Building Resilience Through Routine

A routine can make healthy habits feel more natural. For instance, if you decide to go for a walk every morning right after breakfast, you are less likely to skip it once it becomes a normal part of your day. Similarly, planning your meals in advance can keep you from grabbing unhealthy snacks when you are hungry and short on time.

Routines provide structure, which can help lower stress and anxiety. When your brain knows what to expect, it can relax a bit more. At the same time, try to keep some flexibility so you do not feel trapped by your schedule. The idea is to find a balance between structure and spontaneity.

## Handling Stress in a Healthy Way

Stress is a normal part of life, but it can become harmful if not managed properly. Healthy habits can keep your stress levels in check, but there are other strategies, too:

- **Identify Stress Triggers**: Notice which situations or people cause you the most stress. This awareness helps you prepare and set boundaries when possible.

- **Breathing Techniques**: When stress flares up, slow, deep breaths can calm your nervous system. Inhale slowly for four counts, hold for a moment, then exhale for four counts.
- **Guided Relaxation**: You can find guided relaxation or visualization exercises online. These practices lead you through calm images and settings to help ease tension in your mind and body.

Developing ways to handle stress now will help you later, especially when life becomes more complicated. Remember, it is normal to feel anxious or overwhelmed sometimes. The goal is to respond to it in a way that does not harm your long-term well-being.

## Healthy Social Connections

Your relationships can affect both your physical and mental health. Spending time with people who uplift and respect you can lower stress and boost positivity. On the other hand, toxic relationships can drain you emotionally and even physically.

Try to build a circle of support. This might include friends, family, coworkers, or neighbors. Social connections can also come from community groups, places of worship, or volunteer activities. Being around others who share your interests can create a sense of belonging.

## Avoiding Self-Neglect

While focusing on healthy habits, be cautious about falling into the trap of self-neglect. Sometimes we get so busy taking care of others or fulfilling responsibilities that we forget to look after ourselves. Self-neglect can lead to burnout, low moods, and illness.

If you notice that you are constantly putting your needs last, make a conscious decision to do at least one kind act for yourself daily. It could be as simple as making a cup of tea and enjoying it in silence, or it could be planning a weekend getaway. These small breaks remind you that your well-being is important.

## Finding Joy in Movement

Exercise does not have to feel like a chore. If you force yourself into workouts you hate, you might dread being active. Instead, explore different activities to see what makes you happy: it could be hiking, dancing, yoga, or even jumping rope. Some people find joy in group sports or classes, while others prefer exercising alone. By linking exercise to fun and fulfillment, you are more likely to make it a lasting habit.

## Listening to Your Body

Everybody is different, so be mindful of how your own body responds to various foods, activities, and rest. For example, some people do great with early morning workouts, while others prefer evenings. Some might thrive on three balanced meals a day, while others feel better with smaller, more frequent snacks. Experiment and see what helps you feel most energetic and emotionally stable.

If you suspect that certain foods or habits are making you feel unwell, you may want to keep a simple log of your daily routine and note how you feel. Over time, patterns might become clear. Always seek advice from a healthcare professional if you have ongoing concerns or conditions.

## Incorporating Gratitude

One mental habit that can boost overall health is gratitude. This does not need to be complicated. Simply take a moment each day to acknowledge what you are thankful for. It could be something big, like a supportive friend, or something small, like a tasty meal. Gratitude can shift your focus away from stress and toward what is going well in your life. A positive perspective often improves mental health, which, in turn, can encourage healthier physical choices.

## Simplifying Your Environment

Your physical surroundings can impact your well-being. Cluttered or chaotic spaces can increase anxiety. A simple, organized environment can help you feel calm and in control.

- **Decluttering**: Try to remove items you no longer need or want. Donate or recycle them if possible.

- **Organizing**: Make sure the things you use daily are easy to find. This saves you from frustration and wasted time.
- **Calming Touches**: If you have the space, add elements that bring you peace—like a houseplant, a soft rug, or a favorite piece of art.

Even small changes in your living or working area can make a difference in how you feel. Your environment should support your healthy lifestyle, not make it harder.

## Putting It All Together

Healthy habits for the body and mind are not about quick fixes. They are about long-term changes that become second nature. Each small choice—like drinking a glass of water, taking a short walk, or saying no to something that causes undue stress—adds up over time.

If you ever feel overwhelmed by all the suggestions out there, come back to basics:

1. **Fuel your body** with nutritious foods.
2. **Move regularly** in ways you enjoy.
3. **Sleep well** to allow your body and mind to recharge.
4. **Protect your mental space** with mindfulness, restful breaks, and gratitude.
5. **Stay open** to adjusting what does not work, and keep what does.

You do not need to overhaul your life in one day. Start with one habit at a time, and be patient with yourself. It can take weeks or even months for a new behavior to feel natural.

# Chapter 4: Emotional Healing and Growth

## Introduction

Everyone carries emotional wounds, whether they come from childhood, past relationships, or personal disappointments. These wounds can influence how we see ourselves, how we handle stress, and how we connect with others. Emotional healing is the process of addressing these hurtful experiences, learning from them, and moving forward in a healthier way.

In this chapter, we will explore methods for emotional healing and growth. This is different from simply burying painful memories or pretending everything is fine. True healing involves recognizing your feelings, processing them, and transforming the lessons into new perspectives. This journey can be challenging, but it is worth it. When you heal emotionally, you free up space in your mind for optimism, self-love, and deeper connections with others.

## Recognizing Emotional Wounds

Before you can heal, you need to know what needs healing. Sometimes the source of emotional pain is obvious—like the end of a relationship or a big betrayal. Other times, it might be subtle—a childhood memory that still brings up fear or shame. Reflect on situations that cause you to feel strong emotions, whether anger, sadness, or anxiety. These reactions are often clues that there is an unresolved hurt beneath the surface.

### Common Signs of Unresolved Emotional Pain

- Unexplained mood swings or bursts of anger
- Difficulty trusting others
- Fear of close relationships or emotional intimacy
- Feeling stuck or unable to move on from past events
- Constant negative self-talk tied to a particular memory

If you notice any of these signs, it does not mean something is "wrong" with you. It simply means there might be a part of you that needs attention and compassion.

## Allowing Yourself to Feel

Emotional healing starts with giving yourself permission to feel your emotions, whether they are pleasant or painful. Many of us grow up thinking certain emotions are "bad" or that we should hide them. This leads to bottling everything up, which can grow into anxiety, depression, or physical issues.

Take some quiet time to sit with your feelings. You might cry, feel angry, or become anxious. All these reactions are normal. Let them be, without judging yourself. Imagine you are opening a door to a room full of emotions. You do not have to stay in that room forever, but you need to step inside to see what is there.

## Processing Emotions in a Healthy Way

Feeling your emotions is step one; processing them is step two. Processing means finding a way to understand and release what you are experiencing so it does not stay stuck. Some methods include:

1. **Therapy or Counseling**: A trained professional can provide guidance, tools, and a safe space to explore deep feelings. Talking openly without fear of judgment often speeds up the healing process.
2. **Creative Outlets**: Activities like painting, writing (different from journaling if you prefer creative writing or poetry), or playing music can help express emotions that are hard to put into everyday words.
3. **Support Groups**: Sometimes sharing experiences with people who have gone through similar situations can provide comfort. You realize you are not alone, and you can learn from how others cope.
4. **Meditation and Relaxation**: Gentle meditation techniques can calm the mind, allowing emotions to come forward in a controlled, non-overwhelming way.

Choose whichever method feels most comfortable for you. If you find that one does not work, try another. The goal is to give your emotions a place to go rather than holding them inside.

## Forgiveness and Letting Go

Forgiveness does not mean agreeing with bad behavior or pretending something hurtful never happened. It means deciding that you will no longer let anger and bitterness control your thoughts and actions. Forgiveness can be aimed at others who have hurt you, or it can be aimed at yourself for mistakes you have made.

- **Self-Forgiveness**: Sometimes the hardest person to forgive is yourself. You might carry guilt or shame for past actions. Remember that everyone makes mistakes, and it is through those mistakes that we learn. By forgiving yourself, you acknowledge the error but free yourself from the weight of constant self-blame.
- **Forgiving Others**: This can be tough, especially if the hurt runs deep. However, holding onto resentment can keep you emotionally stuck. When you forgive someone, you do it to release yourself from the ongoing stress and pain. You do not have to invite them back into your life if it is not safe or healthy, but you can let go of the emotional burden.

Forgiveness is a process, not a one-time event. You might think you have forgiven, only to find feelings of anger resurface. Be patient with yourself; each time you recognize these feelings, gently remind yourself of your decision to move forward.

## Learning From Emotional Pain

Painful experiences often come with lessons if we are willing to see them. Maybe a difficult relationship showed you the importance of having clear boundaries. Or a failure taught you to be more prepared next time. By looking for insights in your pain, you shift your perspective from being a victim of circumstances to being someone who grows from challenges.

Questions to ask yourself:

- What did I learn about my needs and limits?
- Are there red flags or warning signs I should watch for next time?
- Did this situation reveal any strength in me I did not know I had?
- How can I use this experience to help others or prevent similar harm in the future?

These questions do not minimize what happened. Instead, they help you use your experience as fuel for personal growth.

## Rewriting Your Story

We all have narratives we tell ourselves about our lives—who we are, what we deserve, and how we got here. Emotional wounds can color these stories in negative ways. You might see yourself as "unlovable," "a failure," or "not worthy of happiness." Part of healing is rewriting these narratives to reflect a more balanced and truthful view.

Try writing a new version of your story, focusing on resilience and hope. For example, if your old story was "I can't trust anyone because I was hurt," your new story might be "I've been hurt before, but I learned to recognize unhealthy patterns. Now I choose relationships that are respectful and caring." Words have power, so be intentional about which ones you use to describe yourself and your journey.

## Setting Emotional Boundaries

After experiencing emotional wounds, you might need to adjust how you interact with people or situations. Setting boundaries is a way to protect your emotional well-being. This can mean:

- Saying "no" to extra responsibilities when you are already feeling overwhelmed
- Limiting contact with someone who drains you or treats you poorly
- Making time for self-care activities without feeling guilty
- Speaking up if someone's behavior crosses a line

Boundaries are not walls to shut people out; they are guidelines that help you feel safe and respected. Over time, these boundaries give you the space to continue healing without getting hurt repeatedly in the same ways.

## Building Emotional Resilience

Resilience is the ability to bounce back from hardships. It does not mean you never feel pain; it means you learn how to recover more quickly. Emotional healing contributes to resilience because it teaches you that you can survive tough times and still come out stronger.

### Ways to Strengthen Resilience

- **Practice Patience**: Healing takes time, so do not rush yourself. Acknowledge that every step, no matter how small, is moving you forward.
- **Maintain Healthy Routines**: As discussed in the previous chapter, good sleep, nutrition, and movement support emotional balance.
- **Focus on Gratitude**: Even in the midst of pain, there can be small good things in your day. Identifying them can help keep your spirits up.
- **Seek Support When Needed**: Talk to friends, family, or professionals when you feel overwhelmed. You do not have to face everything alone.

## Healing Through Connection

Isolation can sometimes feel tempting when you are hurt, but it often slows down healing. Human beings are wired for connection. Sharing your feelings with someone you trust can lighten the load. Even a caring friend who simply listens can make you feel less lonely. If you do not have someone in your immediate circle who is supportive, you might join local support groups or find an online community of people dealing with similar issues.

Being willing to connect also means opening yourself up to the possibility of being hurt again. But healthy connections, over time, can help you see that not every relationship will end in pain. This balance of caution and openness is part of emotional growth.

## Growing Through Self-Compassion

Self-compassion goes beyond self-care. It involves treating yourself with the same kindness and empathy you would offer a loved one who is hurting. Instead of criticizing yourself for past mistakes, you acknowledge that you are human. Instead of hiding your pain, you accept it and seek help.

### Simple Self-Compassion Exercise

1. When negative thoughts arise about something you did or felt, pause.
2. Ask yourself, "What would I say to a friend if she were going through this?"
3. Tell yourself those same comforting, understanding words.
4. Remind yourself that everyone faces struggles, and you are not alone.

Practicing self-compassion regularly can soften harsh self-judgment and boost your emotional well-being. It is not about excusing harmful behaviors; it is about accepting that you can learn and change with kindness.

## Embracing New Possibilities

Healing creates room for new possibilities in your life. When old hurts no longer define you, you might feel freer to pursue dreams or try new activities. This can include exploring different career paths, forming healthier relationships, or finally doing that hobby you always put off.

Sometimes the pain of the past can keep you in a comfort zone, even if it is not truly comfortable. By acknowledging the pain, learning from it, and letting it go, you open yourself up to growth. This does not happen overnight, but each step brings you closer to a future that reflects who you are now, rather than who you were when you were hurt.

## Giving Yourself Time

Deep emotional wounds do not heal instantly. Do not be discouraged if you still feel sad or anxious even after doing a lot of work on yourself. Healing can come in waves; sometimes you feel fine, other times something triggers you, and old feelings resurface. This is normal. A big part of emotional growth is understanding that progress is not always a straight line.

Keep track of your progress to see how far you have come. Maybe you no longer have nightmares about a certain event, or maybe you went a whole week without feeling overwhelmed by sadness. Celebrate these small victories. They show that healing is happening, even if it sometimes feels slow.

## When Professional Help is Needed

While many emotional challenges can be worked through with self-help strategies and support from friends, some wounds are very deep or cause severe distress. If you are experiencing ongoing feelings of hopelessness, intense anxiety, or thoughts of harming yourself or others, reach out to a mental health professional immediately. Therapy or counseling can provide a tailored approach that addresses your specific needs. Seeking help is a sign of strength, not weakness.

# Chapter 5: Effective Communication in Everyday Life

## Introduction

Communication is at the heart of all human relationships. It affects your connections with family, friends, coworkers, and even strangers. Yet many of us struggle to convey our thoughts or needs in a way that leads to understanding. This chapter will help you improve your communication skills so you can express yourself honestly and listen to others with genuine care.

Good communication is not just about talking. It also involves listening actively, interpreting nonverbal cues, handling disagreements, and finding ways to work together. When you communicate effectively, you show respect for yourself and for the people you interact with. This skill can open doors in your personal and professional life, reduce conflicts, and boost your confidence.

## Why Communication Matters

Think about all the areas of your life that depend on communication—romantic relationships, friendships, workplaces, and community events. If you cannot explain how you feel or what you need, misunderstandings tend to multiply. Minor issues can grow into big problems when people talk past each other or avoid talking at all.

Effective communication helps you:

- Build strong bonds based on trust.
- Resolve conflicts before they turn into bigger issues.
- Achieve personal and work-related goals more easily.
- Feel heard and validated as an individual.
- Increase empathy toward others.

Communication is a skill that can be learned and refined. Even if you have felt unheard or misunderstood in the past, you can develop the tools to be a clearer speaker and a more attentive listener.

# The Power of Listening

Many of us think communication is about what we say. In truth, much of it is about how we listen. Active listening means giving your full attention to the speaker. Instead of planning your next reply or letting your mind wander, you focus on understanding what the person is saying.

**Tips for Active Listening**

1. **Maintain Eye Contact (If Culturally Appropriate)**: Looking at the speaker shows you value their words.
2. **Avoid Interrupting**: Let the person finish their thoughts before chiming in.
3. **Ask Clarifying Questions**: If something is unclear, politely ask for more details. For instance, "Could you tell me more about what you meant by that?"
4. **Paraphrase**: Summarize what you heard to confirm understanding, like "So you feel upset because you felt left out, right?" This gives the speaker a chance to correct or confirm your interpretation.

Active listening lets people know you genuinely care about what they are saying. It also reduces confusion because it allows you to check if you heard them correctly. Over time, people may feel safer opening up to you, leading to more honest and respectful conversations.

# Expressing Yourself Clearly

When it is your turn to speak, clarity is key. If you are vague or mix too many points at once, the other person can become lost or defensive. Instead, try to be direct yet kind.

**Focus on One Topic**

Pick the main issue you want to discuss and stay on it. For example, if you are upset about a friend not returning your calls, do not also bring up old gripes about past events unless they are directly related. Sticking to one topic keeps the conversation organized and easier to resolve.

### Use "I" Statements

When expressing your thoughts or feelings, use "I" statements, such as "I feel sad when…" or "I need more time to…" This approach describes how you feel without placing blame. Compare the following:

- "You never listen to me—you are so careless!" vs.
- "I feel ignored when I do not get a response; it makes me think my concerns are not important."

The second approach focuses on your experience rather than attacking the other person's character. This can help the listener feel less defensive.

### Be Specific

Give clear examples rather than general statements. If you say, "You don't help around the house," your partner might have no idea which tasks you mean. If you say, "I would really appreciate it if you could handle the dishes after dinner," that is a specific request. Specificity helps the other person know exactly how to meet your needs.

## Managing Emotions During Conflict

Disagreements happen in every relationship. They are normal. But they can become damaging when tempers flare and harsh words are spoken. Learning to handle conflicts in a calm, constructive way can save relationships and reduce stress.

### Take a Pause

If you notice emotions rising—your voice getting louder, your heart beating faster—it may help to pause. You can say, "I'm feeling upset. Can we take a break and come back to this in 20 minutes?" During that break, try taking a walk, doing some deep breathing, or drinking some water. The goal is to cool off so you can return to the conversation with a clearer mind.

### Focus on the Issue, Not the Person

Instead of name-calling or pointing out character flaws, discuss the specific issue at hand. For instance, if someone forgot to pay a bill on time, focus on how to ensure it is not forgotten next time. Avoid attacking the person's entire character, like "You're always so irresponsible!" That kind of language does not solve the problem and only fuels anger.

### Seek a Win-Win Solution

Try to find a compromise or common ground. Ask the other person, "What do you think would be a fair solution?" Listen to their ideas. Share your own suggestions as well. Aim for an outcome that respects both of your needs. You may not always find a perfect solution, but showing willingness to meet in the middle can build trust and goodwill.

## Nonverbal Communication

Not all communication is verbal. Our bodies, faces, and tone of voice convey messages, often without us realizing it. If your arms are folded and you are scowling, you might seem closed off, even if your words are neutral. Awareness of your body language can make a big difference in how people perceive you.

- **Posture**: Standing or sitting up straight shows confidence and openness.
- **Facial Expressions**: Try to keep your facial muscles relaxed. Tension in your jaw or furrowing your brow can signal stress or anger.
- **Tone of Voice**: A gentle, calm tone usually encourages positive interactions, whereas shouting or sarcasm can instantly raise tensions.

By paying attention to your nonverbal signals, you can ensure your body and words send the same message. You can also become better at reading others' signals, helping you respond more sensitively to their emotions.

## Communicating in Different Settings

Communication styles may need slight adjustments based on the setting. Talking to your boss is not the same as talking to your child. Here are some considerations for three common environments: work, family, and social gatherings.

### Workplace Communication

- **Professionalism**: Even if you have personal conflicts with a coworker, keep your language and tone respectful. Personal insults have no place in a work setting.
- **Clarity in Emails**: Written communication can be tricky because tone is not always clear. Be concise and double-check your words to avoid misunderstandings.
- **Asking for Feedback**: In a job environment, feedback can help you grow. If you are unsure about your performance, politely ask for feedback from your boss or colleagues. Listen openly to their suggestions instead of becoming defensive.

### Family Communication

- **Respect Each Generation**: Family members come from different age groups with different ideas. Listen to them, even if you disagree. You might gain insights or at least show respect for their experiences.
- **Setting Limits**: If certain family members tend to argue about sensitive topics (politics, life choices), learn to steer the conversation gently away when it starts to get heated.
- **Shared Responsibilities**: For household tasks or caregiving, use direct requests rather than complaints. Ask for help in a clear way, and be ready to negotiate who handles which tasks.

### Social Gatherings

- **Inclusivity**: When you are in a group, try to involve quiet members in the conversation by asking them friendly questions.
- **Handling Gossip**: If a conversation turns into harmful gossip, consider changing the subject or politely stating that you would rather not speak negatively about someone.
- **Being Yourself**: Social events can trigger anxiety. Remind yourself that you do not have to impress anyone. Being authentic can lead to more genuine connections.

## The Role of Curiosity

Good communication often involves genuine curiosity about the other person. Instead of assuming you already know what they think, ask questions. People usually appreciate when you show interest in their perspectives or experiences. This curiosity can also help you avoid jumping to wrong conclusions.

- **Open-Ended Questions**: These start with "how," "what," or "why" and encourage deeper answers than just "yes" or "no." For example, "What do you think about the new policy at work?" or "How did you feel about that movie?"
- **Encourage Sharing**: If someone is hesitant to speak, a gentle "I'd really like to hear your thoughts if you're comfortable sharing" can go a long way.

Showing genuine curiosity helps you learn more about others and can reduce tension, especially when discussing sensitive subjects.

## Overcoming Communication Barriers

Communication barriers can be physical (like language differences) or emotional (like fear of judgment). Here are some ways to break down these barriers:

1. **Language Differences**: If someone speaks a different language, use simple words or translation tools if available. Focus on clarity rather than perfect grammar.
2. **Cultural Norms**: Different cultures have different norms for eye contact, personal space, and tone. If you are unsure, a respectful approach with willingness to learn can prevent misunderstandings.
3. **Fear of Rejection**: Sometimes people do not speak up because they fear negative responses. Overcoming this requires self-confidence (discussed in earlier chapters) and an understanding that disagreement is not always rejection.
4. **Technology Distractions**: Phones and computers can interrupt face-to-face conversations. Set devices aside or turn off notifications when you want to have a meaningful talk.

## Apologizing and Repairing Damage

No one communicates perfectly all the time. We all say or do things we regret. Knowing how to apologize sincerely can repair damaged relationships and rebuild trust.

- **Acknowledge the Mistake**: Be clear about what you did wrong. Instead of saying, "I'm sorry you felt bad," say, "I'm sorry I raised my voice at you."
- **Take Responsibility**: Avoid blaming others for your actions. Show that you understand how your behavior affected them.
- **Make Amends**: If possible, do something to fix the situation. That might mean replacing something broken or dedicating time and energy to correct a misunderstanding.
- **Commit to Change**: Explain what you will do to prevent the same mistake. People appreciate seeing genuine effort to improve.

A heartfelt apology shows maturity and respect. It can help rebuild closeness and demonstrate that you value the relationship enough to admit fault.

## Receiving Criticism

Being on the receiving end of criticism can be tough. Our natural response might be to defend ourselves or lash out. However, learning to handle criticism calmly can turn it into a chance for growth.

1. **Listen Fully**: Let the person finish without interrupting. Even if you disagree, hear them out.
2. **Ask Questions**: Clarify points that are unclear, "Can you give me an example?" or "What would you suggest I do differently?"
3. **Consider the Source**: Is the criticism coming from someone with valid expertise or from someone who often criticizes without reason? Take constructive feedback to heart but ignore baseless insults.
4. **Respond Politely**: If the criticism is valid, thank them for their input and share how you plan to address the issue. If it is not, politely explain your perspective without getting personal or insulting.

Receiving criticism well can impress others and also help you identify areas where you can improve. It does not mean you have to agree with everything said, but staying open-minded can reveal insights you might otherwise miss.

## Communicating Assertively

Being assertive means expressing yourself honestly while respecting the rights of others. It is the middle ground between being passive (never speaking up for yourself) and being aggressive (not caring about other people's feelings).

- **Use a Calm Tone**: Even if you are stating a strong opinion, do it in a measured way.
- **Stand Up for Yourself**: If someone crosses a line—maybe they speak rudely or invade your personal space—state that it is not acceptable. "I'd like you to please not shout at me. Let's continue the discussion calmly."
- **Stay Respectful**: Keep your words free of insults or name-calling. You can be firm and respectful at the same time.

Assertive communication can reduce resentment and misunderstandings because everyone knows where they stand. It also increases self-respect, because you are no longer hiding your real thoughts out of fear.

## Maintaining Ongoing Practice

Communication is not a skill you learn once and master forever. It requires regular practice. You might catch yourself reverting to old habits like interrupting or complaining. That is normal. The goal is to notice these slips and correct them.

- **Reflect After Conversations**: Ask yourself what went well and what could have been better.
- **Seek Feedback**: If you trust someone, ask them how you come across. Be open to their observations.
- **Continue Learning**: Books, workshops, or even online videos on communication techniques can offer fresh insights.

As you become more aware and disciplined in your communication, you will likely see improvements in your relationships and self-confidence. People will appreciate your genuine efforts to understand and be understood.

# Chapter 6: Setting Boundaries and Protecting Your Energy

## Introduction

Everyone has personal limits—ways they want to be treated, how they spend their time, and what makes them feel safe or stressed. Boundaries define these limits. They help you protect your well-being, maintain respect in relationships, and ensure that you are not drained by external demands. For many women, setting boundaries can be challenging due to cultural expectations or fear of conflict, but it is an essential step in self-improvement.

In this chapter, you will learn how to recognize when your boundaries are being crossed, how to communicate those boundaries effectively, and how to protect your energy so you can focus on what really matters. Boundaries do not mean shutting people out entirely; they are about drawing lines that help you feel respected and secure.

## Understanding the Importance of Boundaries

If you have ever felt exhausted after interacting with a certain person or anxious about attending a group event, it could be a sign that your boundaries need adjusting. Without clear limits, you might say "yes" to things you really do not want to do, or tolerate behaviors that harm your mental or emotional health.

Boundaries can cover many areas:

- **Emotional Boundaries**: Deciding how much personal information you share, or the types of emotional support you can offer before you become overwhelmed.
- **Physical Boundaries**: Respecting personal space and deciding who can touch you and in what way (even something as simple as a hug).
- **Time Boundaries**: Determining how you allocate your hours for work, rest, and leisure.
- **Digital Boundaries**: Managing when and how people can reach you online or through your phone.

When you set boundaries, you are taking responsibility for your well-being. This is not about being selfish; it is about self-care. You show others how to treat you, and in turn, you often feel more at peace in your relationships.

## Recognizing When Boundaries Are Lacking

Sometimes, people do not even realize their boundaries are weak until they experience burnout or resentment. Here are some signs you may need stronger boundaries:

- **Constant Fatigue**: You feel mentally or physically drained because you keep saying "yes" to tasks or favors.
- **Frequent Anger or Resentment**: You get irritated with others for crossing lines, but you do not express it directly.
- **Lack of Time for Yourself**: Your schedule is full of commitments for others, leaving little room for personal interests or rest.
- **Feeling Guilty for Saying "No"**: Each time you try to set a limit, you experience overwhelming guilt or fear of displeasing people.
- **Being Taken Advantage Of**: You notice people rely on you to do extra work or give extra support without reciprocation.

These feelings are often signals telling you it is time to step back and reassess.

## Determining Your Boundaries

To set boundaries, you must know what they are. Spend time thinking about which situations make you uncomfortable or stressed. Ask yourself:

1. **What personal values guide me?** (e.g., honesty, respect, family time)
2. **How do I want to be treated by friends, family, or coworkers?**
3. **Which tasks or responsibilities feel too overwhelming to keep taking on?**
4. **How much "alone time" do I need to recharge?**

Being honest with yourself is key. You might discover that you are uncomfortable with something but have been going along with it to keep the peace. Recognizing this feeling is the first step toward making a change.

## Communicating Boundaries Clearly

Just like in effective communication (Chapter 5), clarity is essential here. If people do not know your boundaries, they cannot respect them.

### Use Assertive Language

Say, "I need..." or "I prefer..." For instance, if you need downtime after work, you might state, "I need at least an hour to myself after I get home before discussing the day's events." This is not rude; it is honest. It tells others exactly what you expect.

### Avoid Apologizing Excessively

When setting a boundary, you do not need to say, "I'm sorry, but could you maybe...?" That kind of phrasing weakens your position and suggests that your boundary is optional. Instead, be polite and firm: "I won't be answering work emails after 7 p.m. Thanks for understanding."

### Be Consistent

If you say you will not do something, follow through. For example, if you tell a friend you can only chat until 9 p.m., do not keep texting until midnight. Inconsistency sends mixed messages and can lead people to ignore your boundaries in the future.

## Handling Pushback

Not everyone will accept your boundaries graciously, especially if they benefited from your lack of limits in the past. They might push back or try to guilt-trip you. This is where you have to stand firm.

- **Stay Calm**: Respond with a calm tone. Anger or shouting can escalate the situation.
- **Repeat if Necessary**: Sometimes, you have to restate your boundary multiple times. "I understand you want me to stay longer, but I really have to leave at 6 p.m."
- **Offer Alternatives (If Appropriate)**: If someone's request does not fit within your boundary, you might suggest another option: "I can't meet

you today, but I'm free tomorrow afternoon." This shows you are not rejecting them completely—you are just protecting your limits.
- **Accept Their Reaction**: They might be upset or disappointed. You cannot control how others feel. Your job is to maintain your well-being while still being respectful.

Pushback can be tough emotionally, but over time, people who truly value you will adjust. If someone does not respect your repeated boundaries, it might be a sign of a relationship that no longer supports your growth.

## Protecting Your Energy

Boundaries are not just about saying "no." They are also about how you invest your mental and emotional energy.

### Identify Energy Drains

Think about the people or situations that leave you feeling exhausted. Is it a friend who constantly complains? A colleague who expects you to do their work? Sometimes, just becoming aware of these drains can help you manage them better.

### Limit Exposure

If it is possible, reduce the time you spend in draining environments. You do not have to cut people off entirely, but you might see them less often or set a limit on how long you interact. This can be as simple as scheduling a one-hour coffee date instead of three hours at their house.

### Prioritize Self-Care

Self-care is the counterpart to boundary-setting. When you free up time and mental space by saying "no" to certain demands, you can invest that energy in activities that renew you—like hobbies, rest, or learning something new. Protecting your energy means recognizing you have a limited amount of time and emotional capacity. Spend it wisely.

## Dealing with Guilt

Feeling guilty is a major obstacle in setting boundaries. You may worry you are letting people down or coming across as unkind. However, constantly ignoring your own limits is not kindness—it is self-neglect. Remember, you can still help others in ways that do not deplete you. You can still show compassion without burning out.

If guilt creeps in, remind yourself:

1. **Your needs matter**: Caring for yourself allows you to be at your best for the people who rely on you.
2. **Boundaries are healthy**: They do not indicate selfishness; they signal self-respect.
3. **No one can please everyone**: Trying to meet everyone else's expectations is a recipe for exhaustion and unhappiness.

Reframing your thoughts can ease guilt and help you see boundaries as a form of self-respect.

## Workplace Boundaries

Work environments often require clear boundaries to avoid burnout. Maybe your supervisor expects you to answer emails on weekends, or a coworker frequently offloads tasks onto you. Here are some tips:

- **Clarify Expectations**: Politely check with your boss about after-hours communication. Sometimes, they may not realize they are intruding on your personal time.
- **Delegate or Speak Up**: If a coworker assigns you extra work, calmly explain your current workload and discuss what can be prioritized or shared.
- **Take Breaks**: Legally, you often have the right to breaks. Make sure you use them. If you must eat lunch at your desk, at least step away for a quick moment of quiet.

Healthy workplace boundaries not only protect your well-being but can also improve performance by preventing overwhelm and resentment.

## Family Boundaries

Family bonds can be strong but also complicated. You might feel obligated to meet every family request, even when it drains you. Or you might struggle to express your discomfort with certain behaviors.

- **Discuss Roles and Responsibilities**: In a household, clarify who handles which chores or errands. This avoids confusion or arguments later.
- **Handle Sensitive Topics**: If certain subjects (like politics or personal life choices) always lead to fights, set a boundary: "I'd rather not talk about that today." Repeat as needed.
- **Respect Your Own Privacy**: Just because someone is family does not mean they are entitled to know everything about your life. It is okay to keep some matters private.

These boundaries can help you remain close to your family without feeling smothered or stressed.

## Social Boundaries

Friendships and social circles also require boundaries. A friend might always invite you to late-night parties when you need sleep, or constantly call you to vent when you have no emotional energy left.

- **Time Limits**: If you love your friend but find the constant partying draining, be upfront: "I'll join you until 10 p.m., then I have to go home to rest."
- **Emotional Availability**: If you cannot handle your friend's problems at the moment, express empathy but let them know you need some space. You can say, "I understand you're going through a hard time, but I'm currently overwhelmed. Maybe we can chat next week when I'm more able to support you."
- **Social Media**: Online interactions can also be draining. If someone constantly messages you or tags you in posts, set boundaries on response times. You do not have to be available 24/7.

Healthy friendships usually adapt to these boundaries. If someone reacts with anger or refuses to acknowledge your limits, it might be worth reassessing that friendship.

## Overcoming Fear and Anxiety Around Boundaries

It is normal to feel nervous about setting boundaries, especially if you have been accommodating others for a long time. You might worry about conflict, rejection, or being seen as "difficult."

**Practical Steps**

1. **Start Small**: Pick one boundary to set—maybe turning off your phone for an hour a day—and gradually build confidence.
2. **Rehearse**: If you have to confront someone about a boundary issue, practice what you will say beforehand.
3. **Celebrate Success**: Each time you set a boundary and stick to it, acknowledge that achievement. This positive reinforcement will motivate you to continue.

Facing conflict is sometimes part of boundary-setting, but healthy conflict can lead to deeper understanding and more respectful relationships.

## Long-Term Benefits of Boundaries

Establishing and maintaining boundaries has lasting positive effects. You might notice:

- **Less Stress**: You have fewer situations that leave you feeling resentful or overburdened.
- **Stronger Relationships**: People learn to value you and your time. Mutual respect often grows.
- **More Personal Growth**: With your energy protected, you can spend time on self-improvement, hobbies, or educational opportunities.
- **Better Self-Esteem**: Knowing you can stand up for yourself builds confidence.

These benefits compound over time, creating a healthier, more balanced life.

## When Boundaries Are Violated

Despite your best efforts, some individuals may continue to cross your boundaries. If this happens repeatedly, you have to decide what further action is needed. That might mean reducing contact, seeking mediation (in serious cases), or ending the relationship if it is causing significant harm.

You are not obligated to keep people in your life who repeatedly disrespect you. While cutting ties can be painful, it might be necessary for your emotional safety. Remember that respecting yourself is just as important as being kind to others.

## Reviewing and Adjusting Boundaries

Boundaries are not carved in stone. They may evolve as your life changes. A boundary that once made sense might become too restrictive, or you might realize a certain area needs stronger limits.

Check in with yourself periodically:

- **Do I still feel good about this boundary?**
- **Have my priorities shifted, requiring new limits?**
- **Is there an area of my life where I feel used or disrespected?**

Adjusting boundaries as needed keeps them relevant and aligned with your current circumstances.

# Chapter 7: Overcoming Fear and Anxiety

## Introduction

Everyone experiences fear and anxiety at some point. You might feel a knot in your stomach before a big presentation or find yourself unable to sleep because your mind keeps racing with "what if" questions. While these emotions are part of being human, they can become overwhelming if not managed properly. The good news is that you can learn to cope with fear and anxiety in healthier ways, turning these feelings into signals for growth rather than barriers to a fulfilling life.

This chapter will explore the nature of fear and anxiety, why they sometimes take hold, and how to handle them so they do not control you. We will discuss practical strategies you can apply right away. Remember, overcoming fear and anxiety is not about never feeling them again—it is about learning to respond calmly and confidently when they arise.

## Understanding Fear and Anxiety

Fear is usually a response to a real or immediate threat. For example, if you see a snake slithering toward you, fear signals your body to either fight, flee, or freeze. This is your body's natural survival system at work. Anxiety, on the other hand, often appears when you think about future threats or possibilities that might not even come true. You could be worried about failing an exam, losing a job, or getting sick. While anxiety can be useful if it motivates you to prepare, it can also become draining if it is constant or exaggerated.

### The Physical Side

Both fear and anxiety trigger physical reactions: a faster heartbeat, sweaty palms, tense muscles, or a rush of adrenaline. These reactions are normal. They are meant to help you deal with danger. However, if your body stays in this state too often—like when anxiety becomes chronic—it wears you down. You might experience headaches, stomach issues, fatigue, or trouble sleeping.

## The Emotional Side

Fear and anxiety can produce strong emotions such as dread, panic, or a sense of being trapped. Over time, these feelings can affect your self-esteem and relationships if they prevent you from doing things you care about. You might avoid social situations out of fear of embarrassment or pass up new job opportunities because you are anxious about failing.

## Recognizing the Signs

The first step to overcoming fear and anxiety is recognizing when they happen. Sometimes, you might feel a vague sense of worry without knowing the exact cause. Other times, the fear may be tied to a clear situation like public speaking or flying.

Ask yourself:

- **When did this fear or worry first start?**
- **Do certain situations or thoughts trigger it?**
- **How does my body feel when I am afraid or anxious?**

Journaling can help you notice patterns. Write down the times you feel anxious, what you were doing, and what you were thinking. Over days or weeks, you might see that specific events or thoughts trigger your anxiety more than others. This understanding is crucial for dealing with it effectively.

## Changing Unhelpful Thoughts

Much of anxiety arises from unhelpful thinking patterns. For instance, you may jump to the worst possible conclusion ("If I speak up at the meeting, everyone will laugh at me.") or assume you cannot handle what might come your way ("I am not strong enough to handle a new project.").

### Thought Replacement

Once you catch yourself having these negative thoughts, try to replace them with more balanced ones:

- **Negative Thought**: "I will fail this job interview."

- **Balanced Thought**: "I have prepared for this interview, and if things do not go as planned, I can learn from the experience and apply again somewhere else."

This does not mean ignoring real challenges. Rather, it means telling yourself that you can handle those challenges, instead of automatically assuming the worst.

### Realistic Expectations

Fear often grows when you set unrealistic standards. If you expect yourself never to make mistakes, you might feel constant anxiety. Recognize that mistakes and setbacks are part of life. When you accept this, the pressure eases because you know a misstep does not define you.

## Practical Techniques for Calming Down

When fear or anxiety strikes, it helps to have a toolbox of strategies to lower your stress levels.

1. **Deep Breathing**
   Slowly inhale through your nose for a count of four, hold for a second, then exhale through your mouth for a count of four. Focus on your breath. This sends your brain a message to relax.
2. **Progressive Muscle Relaxation**
   Tense and then relax different muscle groups in your body, one by one. Start with your toes and move upward to your head. This method grounds you in the present and releases physical tension.
3. **Grounding Exercises**
   Focus on your surroundings: notice five things you see, four things you can touch, three things you can hear, two things you can smell, and one thing you can taste. This technique helps pull your mind away from worries by anchoring you in the present moment.
4. **Visualizing a Calm Space**
   Close your eyes and imagine a place where you feel safe, like a beach or a forest. Picture the details: the sounds, the scents, the colors. This mental image can calm your nerves and shift your focus away from fear.
5. **Positive Self-Talk**
   Reassure yourself, saying things like, "I am safe right now," or "I can

handle this." Affirmations remind you that you have the ability to get through the situation.

Try different methods to see what works best. You might use one or combine a few. Over time, you will develop a personalized toolkit to manage fear and anxiety effectively.

## Facing Your Fears Gradually

Avoiding fear can make it grow larger in your mind. A common method to lessen fear is called "gradual exposure." Instead of jumping right into the scariest situation, you build up to it step by step.

For instance, if you are afraid of public speaking:

1. Practice giving a short talk at home, just to yourself.
2. Then, speak in front of a close friend or family member.
3. Next, join a small group discussion.
4. Finally, work up to speaking in front of a larger audience.

Each step helps you realize your fear can be handled. The more you face a fear in controlled ways, the less power it has over you.

## Developing a Support System

You do not have to deal with fear and anxiety alone. Friends, family, and professionals can offer insight and encouragement. Share your feelings with people you trust. This not only relieves emotional burden but also helps others understand and support you better.

### Professional Help

If fear or anxiety is severe, consider talking to a counselor or therapist. They can teach you specialized techniques, such as cognitive-behavioral therapy (CBT), to manage anxious thoughts. Therapy is not a sign of weakness; it shows you care enough about your well-being to seek guidance.

## Lifestyle Choices That Reduce Anxiety

Certain daily habits can keep your mind more balanced:

- **Exercise**: Physical activity releases chemicals that improve mood and reduce stress. This can be as simple as a 20-minute walk.
- **Healthy Diet**: Sugary or highly caffeinated foods can spike anxiety levels. Aim for balanced meals that keep your blood sugar steady.
- **Adequate Sleep**: Lack of rest worsens worry and weakens your ability to cope. Strive for 7–9 hours of sleep nightly if you can.
- **Mindful Activities**: Practices like gentle yoga or simple meditation can make your mind calmer and more focused.

By supporting your body with healthy habits, you create a stable base to handle stressful thoughts and situations.

## Accepting Uncertainty

A big part of anxiety comes from wanting to control every outcome. Life, however, is filled with uncertainties—health, relationships, finances, and more. Trying to predict and manage everything is exhausting. Instead, learn to accept that some things are beyond your control. You can plan and prepare, but ultimately, life may take unexpected turns.

Acceptance does not mean giving up. It means acknowledging reality so you can focus your energy on what you can change and let go of what you cannot. This shift in attitude can bring a surprising sense of peace.

## Building Resilience

Resilience is the ability to bounce back from challenges. When you face fear and anxiety head-on, you build resilience. Each time you conquer a small worry or survive a stressful event, you gather evidence that you are capable. This new confidence can then be applied to other areas of your life.

### Self-Compassion

Be kind to yourself if things do not go perfectly. Self-compassion means treating yourself as you would treat a dear friend. If you stumble or feel overwhelmed, remind yourself that growth is a process. Negative self-talk only feeds anxiety. Encouraging words feed resilience.

## Celebrating Progress

Overcoming fear and anxiety is a journey, not a one-time event. As you practice new coping methods, keep track of your progress:

- Did you manage to drive on the highway without feeling panicked this time?
- Did you volunteer to speak up in a meeting?
- Did you manage to replace a negative thought with a more balanced one?

Celebrate these wins, no matter how small. Each victory shows you can face challenges and handle them better than before.

## Knowing Your Limits

While facing fears can be beneficial, it is also important to recognize when you have had enough for the day. Pushing yourself too hard can backfire. Balance courage with self-care. If something is too overwhelming, step back, regroup, and try again later.

## Finding Meaning in Fear

Sometimes, fear can guide you toward areas where you need to grow. If you are terrified of trying a new hobby or speaking up for yourself, that might mean these actions can help you expand your comfort zone. In this sense, fear acts like a compass, pointing you to places where you can evolve. While it is not always easy, viewing fear as a teacher can make it less intimidating.

# Chapter 8: Finding Balance and Managing Stress

## Introduction

Life can feel like a juggling act—work demands, family responsibilities, personal goals, social events, and more. At times, you may wonder how you can possibly keep all the balls in the air without burning out. The answer often lies in finding balance and managing stress in ways that suit your unique needs. Stress itself is not always bad; a moderate amount can push you to grow. But when stress becomes chronic, it can harm your physical health, emotional well-being, and relationships.

In this chapter, we will explore how to identify sources of stress, create a balanced lifestyle, and develop long-lasting strategies to handle pressure. Remember, the goal is not to eliminate all stress—that is impossible—but to manage it effectively so it does not control you.

## Understanding Stress

Stress is your body's response to any demand, whether positive or negative. Getting married, starting a new job, or even planning a vacation can be stressful, even though they are often happy events. On the other hand, deadlines, health issues, and financial worries can bring a type of stress that weighs you down.

**Acute vs. Chronic Stress**

- **Acute Stress** is short-term. It might flare up when you have to give a speech, then fade once the event is over.
- **Chronic Stress** lasts longer. It could come from ongoing situations such as a toxic workplace or financial struggles that do not have an easy solution. Chronic stress can take a toll on your body, leading to fatigue, insomnia, or health problems like high blood pressure.

# Identifying Your Stress Triggers

The first step to managing stress is figuring out what triggers it. Everyone has different triggers, and sometimes they are not obvious. Some people find driving in traffic stressful, while others hardly notice it.

**Self-Reflection**

Take a moment to list the events or situations that regularly raise your stress level. These might include:

- A high-pressure job
- Unresolved conflicts with loved ones
- Lack of personal time
- Health concerns
- Social obligations you do not enjoy

Once you identify these triggers, you can start making plans to address them. This might involve better time management, seeking help for conflicts, or learning to say "no" to invitations that do not truly interest you.

## The Art of Prioritizing

When life feels too hectic, it often means you are trying to do too much at once or spending energy on tasks that do not really matter. Prioritizing means deciding which tasks are truly important and focusing on them first.

- **Create a To-Do List**: Write down everything you need to do, from major projects to small errands.
- **Rank Them**: Mark which tasks are urgent, which are important, and which are neither urgent nor important.
- **Delegate or Drop**: If a task is not important or can be handled by someone else, consider letting it go or asking for help.

This method helps you use your time wisely. It also reduces the mental burden of trying to hold every single task in your head.

## Scheduling Breaks and Downtime

In the rush of daily life, you might feel like you cannot afford to take breaks. But consistent, small breaks can keep you more productive in the long run. If you work at a desk, stand up every hour or so. Stretch, get a glass of water, or simply look out a window and clear your mind. These micro-breaks help reset your brain and prevent burnout.

### The Power of "Me Time"

Setting aside at least a little time each day just for yourself is crucial. You can read a book, take a bath, do a hobby, or simply sit quietly without distractions. This personal time is not a luxury; it is a necessary part of stress management. If your day is very busy, try waking up 10 minutes earlier or using part of your lunch break to unwind.

## Healthy Boundaries with Time and Energy

Setting boundaries (as discussed in Chapter 6) can greatly reduce stress. When you protect your time and energy, you avoid being pulled in too many directions. For instance, if coworkers often ask you to do more than your fair share, kindly but firmly say, "I'm already at capacity, so I can't take on more tasks right now." This may feel uncomfortable at first, but it prevents constant overload.

## Coping Methods for High-Stress Situations

Even with good planning, stress can hit hard—like when a family member falls ill or you are given a tight deadline at work. Here are some effective coping strategies:

1. **Break Tasks Into Smaller Steps**
   A big project can feel crushing, but splitting it into smaller chunks makes it more manageable. Celebrate each step you complete.
2. **Focus on What You Can Control**
   Sometimes, certain parts of a stressful situation are outside your control, such as company layoffs or a sudden illness. Direct your energy toward what you can change, like updating your resume or arranging medical support.

3. **Stay Organized**
   Clutter and disorganization can add to stress. Keep your workspace tidy, use calendars or apps to track appointments, and create routines that make tasks simpler.
4. **Reach Out for Support**
   Do not be afraid to let friends, family, or professionals know you are struggling. A supportive conversation can lighten the emotional load, and loved ones might offer help or solutions you have not thought of.

## The Role of Mindset in Stress Management

Your mindset—the way you think about challenges—matters. If you see stress as a sign that life is falling apart, it can feel more overwhelming. But if you view stress as a natural part of growth or an opportunity to learn, your body might handle it better.

### Flexible Thinking

Being mentally flexible means adjusting your perspective when faced with setbacks. For instance, if your vacation plans fall through, you could spend days feeling upset, or you could see it as a chance to explore local attractions or take a staycation. Flexibility in how you respond helps reduce the emotional weight of disappointments.

## Simple Stress-Reducing Techniques

Like dealing with fear and anxiety (Chapter 7), stress management often involves having a go-to list of strategies for immediate relief.

- **Deep Breathing**: Take slow, controlled breaths to calm your nervous system.
- **Quick Exercise**: A short walk, a few jumping jacks, or stretches can release tension.
- **Music Therapy**: Listening to soothing music can distract your mind from worries.
- **Guided Imagery**: Picture a peaceful scene in your mind—a blooming meadow or a gentle ocean wave—to settle racing thoughts.

Experiment to find what works best for you. Everyone is different, so a technique that helps your friend may not be as effective for you.

## Balancing Work and Personal Life

Many women struggle with balancing career ambitions and personal or family life. You may feel pressured to excel at work while also being a perfect mother, daughter, partner, or friend. This pressure can escalate stress levels if not addressed.

### Setting Clear Work Hours

If your job allows it, decide on clear start and end times. Try not to check work emails late into the evening. Communicate these boundaries to your coworkers or boss, so they understand when you are off-limits for work tasks. Sticking to these times protects you from being "on the clock" 24/7.

### Family Agreements

Discuss household chores and responsibilities with the people you live with. Make a fair plan so you are not carrying all the household tasks alone. A shared calendar can also help coordinate schedules without confusion.

## Learning to Say "No"

Saying "yes" to every request can quickly overload your schedule. Sometimes, you might worry about disappointing people or missing out on opportunities. But trying to do everything often leads to burnout. Practicing a polite "no" when you are already stretched thin can be a form of self-care. You are not rejecting the person—you are valuing your limits so you can be fully present for the things you do commit to.

## Avoiding Perfectionism

Striving for excellence is different from seeking perfection. Perfectionism sets unrealistic standards and can make you overly critical of yourself and others. This creates ongoing stress because you are never fully satisfied. Instead, aim for doing your best within reasonable limits. Ask yourself if certain tasks truly require perfection or if "good enough" is acceptable.

## Time for Fun and Relaxation

All work and no play leads to exhaustion. Schedule fun activities that make you laugh or feel creative—this could be a dance class, watching a comedy show, playing board games, or trying a new recipe. Relaxation is not a waste of time; it recharges you so you can return to your tasks with renewed energy.

## Physical Health and Stress

Chronic stress can harm your physical health. That is why it is important to support your body with good habits:

- **Nutrition**: Fueling your body with balanced meals keeps your energy stable.
- **Exercise**: Regular movement helps release tension and stabilizes mood.
- **Sleep**: A well-rested mind deals with stress more effectively.
- **Hydration**: Dehydration can worsen fatigue and irritability.

While these may sound like general health tips, they have a direct impact on how stressed you feel. Taking care of your body is part of taking care of your mind.

## Digital Detox

Constant notifications, emails, and social media updates can keep you in a state of alert. Consider setting specific times each day to check your phone or social apps. Turn off non-essential notifications. If possible, avoid scrolling through your phone right before bed or first thing in the morning. A small digital detox can calm your mind and reduce background stress.

## Knowing When to Seek Help

Stress can sometimes become too much to handle alone. If you experience persistent anxiety, severe mood swings, trouble sleeping, or a lack of enjoyment in activities you used to love, it might be time to consult a mental health professional. Therapists and counselors can offer guidance tailored to your situation. Seeking help is a sign of strength, not weakness.

## Building a Support Network

A strong network of friends, family members, or support groups can be invaluable for stress relief. Even a short chat over coffee or a phone call can remind you that you are not alone. Look for local groups or online communities focused on similar interests or challenges. Helping others in these communities—by offering an encouraging word or sharing tips—can also lighten your own stress.

## Monitoring Your Progress

Take time every few weeks to see how you are doing with stress management:

- Have you been able to say "no" to extra tasks when needed?
- Are you taking regular breaks and personal time?
- Do you feel more balanced, or are you still rushing through every day?

Adjust your approach based on what you find. If you are still feeling overwhelmed, consider other strategies or talk to someone you trust for fresh ideas.

# Chapter 9: Personal Values and Life Purpose

## Introduction

You have spent time understanding yourself, building confidence, and learning to manage stress. Now, it is worth digging deeper into why you do the things you do and how they connect to the bigger picture of your life. This is where personal values and life purpose come in. Values are the core beliefs that guide your decisions, while purpose gives your life direction and meaning. When you live in harmony with your values and purpose, you often feel more fulfilled and less conflicted.

It is normal to feel unsure about your purpose. Some people discover it early; others find it later after many life experiences. Either way, your purpose is not set in stone. It can shift as you learn new things, meet new people, and face new challenges. In this chapter, we will explore ways to identify your personal values and discover or refine your life purpose in a way that makes sense to you.

## Understanding Personal Values

Your values influence how you see the world and make decisions. They can stem from your upbringing, culture, personal experiences, or even the qualities you admire in others. Examples of common values include honesty, compassion, loyalty, independence, creativity, adventure, family, or personal growth.

### Why Values Matter

- **Decision-Making**: Knowing your values helps you decide what to say "yes" or "no" to. For instance, if you value creativity, you might choose a hobby or a career path that lets you be imaginative.
- **Inner Peace**: When you act according to your values, you feel more at ease because your actions match who you are. On the other hand, going against your values can create guilt or discomfort.

- **Guidance During Hard Times**: Values serve as a compass when life becomes confusing or stressful. You can ask yourself, "Which choice here is most in line with my deepest beliefs?"

## Discovering Your Values

If you have never thought much about your values, you can start by reflecting on these questions:

1. **Who or what inspires me?**
   Think about role models or experiences that left a strong impression. What qualities did those people or events show?
2. **What qualities do I want to see in my relationships?**
   Maybe you value loyalty in friendships or honesty in family members. This often reveals which values matter most to you personally.
3. **When do I feel most fulfilled?**
   Recall moments when you felt truly satisfied or proud. What values were present at those times?
4. **What traits do I admire in others?**
   Perhaps you respect people who are brave, empathetic, or dedicated to a cause. These admired traits can hint at your own core values.

Write down any words or ideas that come to mind, like "trust," "kindness," "freedom," or "growth." Then choose the top five or six that resonate most strongly. Do not worry if your list changes later. You are allowed to evolve as you learn more about yourself.

## Living According to Your Values

It is one thing to know your values, but it is another to apply them daily. This process involves making conscious choices that line up with what you believe in. For instance, if generosity is important to you, you might volunteer, donate, or simply look for ways to help neighbors or friends in need. If health is a core value, you will prioritize exercise and healthy eating.

Sometimes, living your values means changing old habits. If you claim to value respect but find yourself being rude when stressed, that is a signal to practice better communication (discussed in Chapter 5). If you value family but always work late, you might decide to carve out dedicated family time. Each step you take to honor your values makes you feel more consistent and proud of who you are.

## Dealing with Conflicts

There may be times when values clash. Maybe you value both stability and adventure. This can create tension when you yearn for something new but do not want to risk losing the comfortable life you have built. Or you might value loyalty to family but also want independence to live your own way. Recognize these conflicts as natural. In such cases, look for a middle ground or decide which value holds priority in that specific situation.

- **Example**: You receive a job offer that pays more (value: financial stability) but requires you to move far from family (value: close relationships). You might weigh the pros and cons or see if remote work is an option. You could plan regular visits or video calls to stay connected. The final decision will depend on which value feels most urgent to honor at this point in your life.

## The Concept of Life Purpose

While values guide daily decisions, purpose is a broader sense of direction. It answers the question, "Why am I here?" or "What do I want my life to contribute to the world?" Purpose can be tied to your career, personal growth, community service, creative expression, or any combination of these. Finding purpose does not mean you must do something grand or world-changing. It can be as simple as bringing joy to your family or neighborhood.

## Finding Your Purpose

Discovering your life purpose is a process. Some approaches include:

1. **Reflect on Your Passions**
   Passions are things you love doing, even if they are hard. They could be hobbies, social causes, or skills you enjoy developing. Ask yourself what you would do even if you were not paid for it.
2. **Recall Challenges You Have Overcome**
   Sometimes, a life struggle can point you toward a purpose. If you faced a

tough situation—like battling an illness or dealing with loss—you might feel called to help others with similar problems.
3. **Think About Your Unique Strengths**
Each person has a set of skills and talents. Maybe you are great at comforting people, organizing events, or teaching kids. Your purpose may revolve around using these natural gifts to benefit yourself and others.
4. **Listen to What People Praise You For**
Friends and family often notice your best qualities. If they frequently thank you for being a good listener, a dedicated volunteer, or a talented artist, pay attention. Their feedback can guide you toward areas where you truly shine.

## Testing and Adjusting

You do not have to find your life purpose overnight. Consider trying different experiences to see what resonates. Volunteer for a local charity. Start writing a blog about a topic you love. Take a short course in something that intrigues you. Each step you take provides feedback about what feels right and what does not.

If you try something and discover it is not for you, that is still useful information. You learn about what does not fit your life purpose, allowing you to move on and try something else. Purpose is discovered through action and reflection, not through waiting for a lightning bolt of clarity.

## Combining Values and Purpose

Ideally, your purpose should be deeply linked to your values. For example, if you value compassion, your purpose might involve caring for others in some way—perhaps through counseling, teaching, or community service. If you value creativity, your purpose could revolve around writing, art, or designing innovative solutions for problems you care about.

Whenever you feel uncertain about your path, return to the values you identified. Ask yourself, "Does this path allow me to express my core values?" If the answer is yes, you are likely on the right track. If not, you can adjust your direction.

## Balancing Real-Life Responsibilities

Even when you have a clear purpose, life can be complicated. You may have bills to pay, children to raise, or other duties that seem unrelated to your personal calling. Keep in mind that purpose does not erase practical needs. Instead, it guides how you navigate them.

- **Example**: Suppose you feel your purpose is to help homeless animals. You might have a full-time job that pays your bills but volunteer at an animal shelter on weekends. Or you could look for a way to transition into a related career, like working for an animal rescue organization, if that becomes financially feasible.

Small steps still honor your purpose, even if you cannot devote all your time to it immediately. The key is integrating your calling into your life in realistic ways.

## Overcoming Obstacles

Pursuing a meaningful life path often involves challenges. You might face financial constraints, lack of support from others, or your own fears of failure. Here are a few ways to handle obstacles:

1. **Set Smaller Goals**: Break a big dream into steps. Focus on what you can do now rather than feeling overwhelmed by the entire journey.
2. **Seek Mentors and Allies**: Find people who share your passion or have walked a similar road. They can offer guidance, support, or resources you might not have known about.
3. **Keep Learning**: Whether your purpose involves a skill (like art) or a cause (like social justice), continuous learning helps you grow. This might involve formal education, online research, or joining local groups.
4. **Practice Resilience**: When things go wrong, remind yourself why you started. Reflect on how far you have come. Failures and detours can strengthen your resolve if you choose to see them as lessons.

## Staying True to Yourself

Living a purposeful life does not mean you will never experience doubt or worry. Society, friends, or family may sometimes question your choices. They might have different values or see success in ways that clash with your idea of purpose.

Stay open to feedback, but also trust your inner voice. If you feel certain that a path aligns with your values, allow yourself room to pursue it, even if others do not fully understand at first.

## Celebrating Personal Wins

Each time you take a step that aligns with your values or brings you closer to your purpose, take a moment to celebrate. These wins could be small, like completing a challenging online course, or bigger, like launching a community project. Recognizing these achievements builds momentum and keeps you motivated. It also reminds you that you are capable of more than you might think.

## Evolving Purpose

Your purpose can grow and shift as you go through life. You might start out passionate about teaching kids, then discover a deeper interest in writing books for them. Or maybe you focus on local community projects in your 20s and later switch to global issues in your 30s or 40s. This is not a sign of inconsistency; it is a sign of growth. Let your purpose evolve naturally as you gain new knowledge and experiences.

## Avoiding Burnout

A strong sense of purpose can sometimes lead to overwork if you push yourself too hard. You might feel so driven to make a difference that you forget to rest or maintain healthy boundaries. Remember the lessons from Chapters 6 (Boundaries) and 8 (Stress Management). Setting limits on your time and energy ensures you can continue pursuing your purpose in a sustainable way. Burning out will only slow you down.

## Purpose Beyond Work

Some people assume that purpose has to tie directly to a career. While that can be true, you can also fulfill your purpose through community service, relationships, spiritual practices, or personal projects. For instance, if you value mentorship, you might volunteer as a youth mentor or help guide new employees at work. Your purpose is not limited to earning money; it is about finding meaning and contribution in all areas of life.

## Reviewing Your Journey

As you continue to reflect on your values and purpose, keep in mind how far you have come. Maybe you used to make decisions without any sense of direction, and now you pause to consider what truly matters. That is growth. Periodically review your journal entries or personal reflections to see patterns. You may realize you are closer to your ideal lifestyle than you thought.

# Chapter 10: Career Growth and Professional Development

## Introduction

For many women, a significant portion of life is spent working, whether in an office, a lab, a studio, or a virtual environment. If your career aligns with your personal values and goals, it can become a source of satisfaction and growth. On the other hand, if your job feels mismatched with who you are, it can lead to stress, burnout, or a sense that something is missing. This chapter focuses on taking charge of your career path in a way that matches your unique blend of abilities, interests, and life aspirations.

Career growth is not just about promotions and salary increases—though those can be important. It also includes professional development, learning new skills, building relationships, and staying adaptable in a world where jobs and technologies change rapidly. By the end of this chapter, you will have concrete ideas on how to shape your professional journey, whether you are just starting out or looking to pivot into a new field.

## Clarifying Your Career Goals

Before making career decisions, it helps to have clear goals. Ask yourself: "What do I want from my work?" Some common answers include:

- **Financial Stability**: Earning enough to support yourself or your family.
- **Creative Expression**: Using your talents to produce art, design, writing, or innovative ideas.
- **Helping Others**: Contributing to a cause, teaching, or improving the community through your profession.
- **Leadership**: Aiming for roles where you can guide teams or influence major decisions.
- **Flexibility**: Having the freedom to work remotely or set your own hours.

You may value more than one of these outcomes, or have an entirely different set of priorities. Try to rank which matters most to you right now. Your ranking might change over time, and that is normal. Having clarity about your present priorities helps guide your decisions about education, job opportunities, and personal development paths.

## Assessing Your Skills and Strengths

Everyone has a mix of talents. Some are obvious, like being good with numbers or excelling at public speaking. Others might be subtler, like empathy, creativity, or problem-solving. Take an honest inventory of your skills:

- **Technical Skills**: For instance, coding, data analysis, graphic design, or proficiency in a second language.
- **Soft Skills**: Communication, teamwork, time management, leadership, or adaptability.
- **Passions**: Subjects or tasks you love engaging with—writing, organizing events, working with children, etc.

If you are unsure about certain abilities, ask for feedback from friends, family, or coworkers. Sometimes they see strengths you overlook. Understanding your skills helps you pinpoint which roles or industries might be a good fit for you.

## Building a Personal Brand

No matter where you work, your personal brand is the reputation or image you cultivate. It is how people perceive you based on your behavior, skills, and contributions. This brand can open doors to new opportunities or help you stand out in a competitive market.

### Elements of a Personal Brand

1. **Professional Image**: Your manner of speaking, dressing, and interacting in professional settings.
2. **Online Presence**: Social media profiles, LinkedIn, or personal websites that showcase your work.
3. **Consistency**: Ensuring your message and values come across the same way, whether in person or online. If you claim to value teamwork, for example, people should see you acting supportively on group projects.

You do not need to become someone else to build a brand. Just highlight the best aspects of your authentic self. Maybe you are known for your attention to detail, or maybe you bring creative insights to every meeting. Let that shine.

## Networking with Purpose

Networking is about building genuine relationships, not just collecting business cards or sending mass invitations on social media. You want connections that can teach you something, share advice, or even become friends or mentors.

- **Be Genuine**: Start by showing curiosity about the other person's work or goals. Offer help when you can, such as sharing a useful resource or introducing them to someone in your circle.
- **Join Groups or Events**: Professional associations, online forums, or local meetups can help you find people with similar interests. This is especially valuable if you are looking to switch fields or learn new skills.
- **Follow Up**: If you meet someone interesting at an event, drop them a short message afterward saying how nice it was to talk. This small effort can set the stage for future collaboration.

## Continuous Learning

In today's fast-changing work world, learning never really ends. New technologies emerge, industries evolve, and job roles shift. If you want to grow in your career, stay curious and open to learning. This could mean:

- Taking online courses or workshops to learn new software, languages, or creative techniques.
- Attending conferences or seminars related to your field.
- Seeking certifications that boost your credibility, like project management or specialized technical skills.
- Asking for challenging tasks at work to stretch your abilities.

Learning does not always happen in a classroom setting. Mentorship or even reading a good book in your field can be just as valuable. Over time, continuous learning sets you apart because you become more adaptable and knowledgeable.

## Career Transitions

Many women change careers at least once in their lifetime. You might shift from teaching to technology, or from corporate jobs to starting your own business. Transitions can be exciting and scary at the same time. Here's how to make them smoother:

- **Do Your Research**: If you want to enter a new field, read about it, talk to people already in it, and figure out what skills are in demand.
- **Start Small**: Volunteer or take part-time projects to gain experience before making a full leap.
- **Highlight Transferable Skills**: Communication, leadership, problem-solving—these skills apply to many fields. Make sure to point them out in your resume or interview.
- **Mentally Prepare**: Transitions often come with uncertainty. Remind yourself of the reasons why you want this change, and acknowledge it is normal to feel nervous.

By taking careful steps, you can explore new directions without feeling overwhelmed. Transitioning can also help you align your career with your evolving values and sense of purpose (as discussed in Chapter 9).

## Overcoming Workplace Barriers

Even today, women can face unique challenges in the workplace—like gender bias, wage gaps, or a lack of representation in leadership roles. While society is slowly changing, you can take steps to empower yourself in the meantime:

- **Build a Support System**: Seek out mentors or peer groups that understand your situation. Having someone who has "been there" can guide you on navigating tough situations.
- **Document Your Achievements**: Keep a record of projects you have completed, challenges you have solved, and any praise you have received. This list helps you negotiate promotions or raises with concrete evidence.
- **Stand Up for Yourself**: If you feel disrespected or overlooked, address the situation in a calm, direct way. This might involve talking to HR or a supervisor. Knowing your rights is important.

- **Work-Life Balance**: Many women juggle professional work and family responsibilities. Discuss flexible schedules or remote options if possible. Clear communication of your needs can lead to better arrangements.

## Goal-Setting and Action Plans

It is easy to daydream about future success but harder to turn that dream into reality without a plan. Set short-term and long-term career goals. For example:

- **Short-Term (3–6 months)**: Update your resume, take an online course, or improve your public speaking skills.
- **Long-Term (1–5 years)**: Aim for a leadership position, start a business, or transition to a new industry.

List out the specific steps for each goal, along with deadlines. This keeps you accountable and helps you track progress. Remember, goals can be adjusted as you learn new information or your priorities change.

## Handling Rejection and Failure

Rejection is part of any growth process. You might apply for a dream job and not get it, or try to pitch an idea that gets turned down. While disappointment hurts, it can also teach you valuable lessons. Ask for feedback if you can. Maybe you need more experience in a certain area or a stronger presentation style. Then use that feedback to improve. Failure does not mean you are unworthy; it is often just a sign that you need to tweak your strategy or timing.

## Negotiation and Self-Advocacy

Many women feel uncomfortable asking for a higher salary or better benefits, but negotiation is a key part of career growth. You deserve fair compensation for the value you bring.

- **Know Your Worth**: Research market salaries for your role. Keep a list of your accomplishments, skills, and the positive feedback you have received.
- **Prepare Your Case**: Before a performance review or salary discussion, practice what you want to say. Have clear examples of your contributions.

- **Stay Confident and Polite**: You can be assertive without being aggressive. Use a calm tone, make eye contact (if the meeting is in person), and state your requests clearly.
- **Consider the Whole Package**: If the company cannot budge on salary, negotiate other perks like extra vacation days, remote work, or professional development funding.

Negotiation is a skill that grows with practice. Each time you advocate for yourself, you are taking charge of your career path.

## Balancing Ambition with Well-Being

Ambition can be a powerful motivator, but beware of burnout (see Chapters 6 and 8). You do not have to sacrifice all your personal time or health to advance in your career. Sometimes, taking a slower path that includes rest, family time, and self-care may lead to a longer-lasting and more satisfying career.

If you start feeling overwhelmed, revisit your boundaries. Remind yourself why you set certain limits on your work hours or workload. A balanced approach often leads to better performance and more creativity over the long haul, because you are not constantly running on empty.

## Celebrating Career Milestones

It is easy to move from one achievement to the next without pausing to celebrate. Yet acknowledging milestones—like completing a big project, earning a promotion, or reaching a sales goal—boosts your morale. It can also energize you for the next challenge. Share your successes with supportive friends or colleagues, and let them share in the joy. Even a small reward, like a nice meal or a day off, can reinforce the positive feelings that come from progress.

## Staying Adaptable

With technology rapidly evolving and industries shifting, adaptability is a prized trait. Stay open to change, whether it is a new project at work or an unexpected job offer. Even if you love your current role, try to keep track of new developments in your field. Read articles, follow thought leaders, or attend webinars to keep your knowledge fresh. Adaptability will make you more confident facing the unknown, because you know you can learn new skills and pivot when needed.

## Leading and Mentoring Others

As you grow in your career, you may have the chance to lead or mentor others. This is not just about telling people what to do; it is about guiding them to find their strengths and succeed. Mentoring can be very fulfilling, especially when you see someone grow because of your support or advice. It also builds your leadership skills—communication, empathy, and the ability to inspire a shared vision.

# Chapter 11: Nurturing Supportive Relationships

## Introduction

No matter how independent or self-reliant you are, relationships play a vital role in your personal growth. Positive connections with others provide emotional support, encouragement, and a sense of belonging. They also offer different perspectives and experiences that can help you see the world in new ways. Unfortunately, not all relationships are supportive—some can be draining or even harmful. Learning to build and maintain positive bonds, while stepping away from those that negatively impact you, is crucial for a balanced and fulfilling life.

In this chapter, we will dive into how to recognize supportive relationships, nurture them over time, and handle challenges that arise. Whether you are focusing on family ties, friendships, romantic partnerships, or new acquaintances, the principles remain largely the same: mutual respect, understanding, trust, and kindness.

## Recognizing Healthy and Supportive Relationships

A supportive relationship is one in which both parties feel valued and heard. This does not mean there are never disagreements; conflict happens in every relationship. What makes a difference is how you deal with those conflicts and whether respect remains even during tough moments.

Key signs of a healthy, supportive relationship:

1. **Mutual Respect**: Both of you honor each other's boundaries and opinions.
2. **Open Communication**: You can express feelings or concerns without fear of harsh judgment or retaliation.
3. **Consistency**: The other person's actions generally match their words; they are not unpredictable in ways that cause you constant anxiety.
4. **Empathy and Understanding**: When problems arise, you both try to see each other's perspective.

5. **Encouragement**: Each of you feels comfortable sharing achievements or goals, knowing the other will cheer you on.

Not every connection will have all these qualities to the same degree, but if a relationship shows most of them consistently, it is likely positive and supportive.

## Building Trust and Emotional Intimacy

Trust is the cornerstone of any close relationship. It grows through honesty, consistency, and a willingness to be vulnerable. Emotional intimacy, on the other hand, goes beyond sharing lighthearted stories; it involves revealing deeper parts of yourself.

- **Honesty**: This includes not only telling the truth but also avoiding half-truths or lies of omission. When you are honest—even about mistakes—you build an environment where the other person feels safe to be honest as well.
- **Reliability**: If you say you will do something, do your best to follow through. Cancelling plans repeatedly or making excuses erodes trust.
- **Vulnerability**: Sharing your fears or dreams can feel risky, but it often deepens closeness. When you show that you trust someone enough to reveal personal thoughts, it encourages them to do the same.

Healthy relationships involve a balance of give and take in these areas. If one person is always vulnerable while the other never opens up, the relationship can feel one-sided.

## Strengthening Family Bonds

Family relationships are sometimes the closest but also the most complicated. They can be a source of deep security or ongoing tension. If your family ties are generally loving, but you still face challenges (like sibling rivalries or generational gaps), open communication is key. Try the following:

1. **Regular Check-Ins**: Whether it is a weekly phone call or monthly family dinner, consistent contact can keep misunderstandings from piling up.
2. **Active Listening**: Make a real effort to understand where family members are coming from, especially if you disagree. Let them speak without interruption.

3. **Shared Activities**: Simple traditions—like cooking together or doing a weekend walk—help maintain closeness.
4. **Healthy Conflict Resolution**: It is okay to take breaks if tempers flare. You can say, "Let me think about this and talk later," instead of forcing a conversation in the heat of the moment.

If certain family members are toxic or disrespectful (see Chapter 6 for boundary-setting advice), it might be necessary to limit your interaction for the sake of your own well-being. Family ties can be strong, but you should never feel obligated to stay in a situation that harms you consistently.

## Cultivating Lasting Friendships

Friends are often the people you choose as your extended family. They can bring joy, shared experiences, and a sense of community. Yet, friendships, like all relationships, require effort and care.

- **Quality Over Quantity**: Having many acquaintances is fine, but close friendships often develop over time as you share experiences and gradually trust each other more.
- **Finding Common Ground**: Friendships often start because of a shared interest, whether it's a hobby, a volunteering project, or a work connection. Build on those commonalities by doing more activities together.
- **Respect Each Other's Growth**: As you move through life, your interests or priorities might change. Strong friendships adapt to these shifts rather than resist them. A friend who truly cares will celebrate your growth, even if it means seeing you a bit less often.
- **Small Gestures Count**: Thoughtful messages or spontaneous gifts can show you care. Sometimes just a text saying, "Thinking of you—hope you're okay," can brighten a friend's day.

Of course, not all friendships are meant to last forever. Some serve a purpose during a specific stage of life. If a friendship becomes draining or toxic, remember that it is okay to step back or end it if needed.

## Healthy Romantic Partnerships

Romantic relationships can bring intense happiness and deep emotional experiences. However, they can also be challenging if built on shaky ground. Supportive romantic partnerships often share traits with other strong relationships—trust, respect, empathy—but with added layers of emotional and sometimes physical intimacy.

- **Shared Values**: While you do not have to agree on everything, having core values in common (like honesty, loyalty, or personal growth) usually fosters stability.
- **Communication About Needs**: Be clear about your emotional and physical needs. Do not assume your partner can read your mind.
- **Respect for Individuality**: Healthy couples support each other's personal goals and interests without insisting on doing everything together.
- **Conflict as Growth**: Disagreements will happen. The important part is how you handle them—aim for problem-solving rather than blame.
- **Mutual Support**: Ideally, both partners encourage each other's successes. One partner's achievements should not threaten the other.

If a romantic partner repeatedly undermines your self-worth, ignores your feelings, or mocks your ambitions, it is a major red flag. A loving relationship should not leave you feeling worse about yourself most of the time.

## Expanding Your Social Circle

Beyond family, friends, and romantic partners, you can build a wider network of supportive acquaintances. This can include coworkers, neighbors, classmates, or fellow members of a hobby group. While these connections may not always become close friendships, they can provide valuable support, ideas, and opportunities for collaboration.

1. **Join Groups or Communities**: Whether it is a hiking club, a book club, or a local volunteer organization, being around people with similar interests can spark new connections.
2. **Be Open**: If you are shy, try taking small social risks—ask a coworker if they want to grab lunch, or strike up a conversation with a fellow volunteer.

3. **Offer Help**: Simple gestures, like helping someone carry boxes or sharing knowledge, can deepen a sense of community. It shows you are willing to contribute, not just receive.
4. **Stay Curious**: Ask people about their interests and experiences. Genuine curiosity often leads to more meaningful conversations.

## Navigating Cultural and Generational Differences

In a diverse society, you may form bonds with people from different backgrounds or age groups. This diversity can enrich your life by exposing you to new traditions, viewpoints, and life lessons. However, misunderstandings can arise when communication styles or expectations differ.

- **Ask Questions Respectfully**: If you do not understand someone's cultural practice, politely ask them to explain, showing genuine interest in learning.
- **Practice Patience**: Sometimes generational gaps lead to different views on technology, social norms, or career paths. Rather than dismissing these views, try to see what you can learn from them—and share your perspective in return.
- **Focus on Shared Values**: Often, underneath surface differences, you might share common values like family, kindness, or self-improvement.

## Maintaining Relationships Through Life Changes

Life events—moving to a new city, changing jobs, getting married, having children, going through a divorce, or losing a loved one—can test even the closest relationships. One person's life shift may alter the dynamics, leaving less time for one another or introducing new conflicts.

- **Communication is Key**: If you are going through a major change, tell the people close to you how you feel and what you need. Maybe you need space, or maybe you need extra support.
- **Adapt Expectations**: When a friend has a newborn, they may not be as available to chat at night. If you move to a new city, old friends might need more planning to stay in touch. Adjusting expectations keeps resentment from building.

## Overcoming Conflict and Misunderstandings

No relationship is without conflict. Healthy conflict can help both people grow, as long as it is approached with respect and an aim to resolve issues rather than "win."

1. **Stay Focused on the Issue**: Avoid bringing up past mistakes that are not directly related.
2. **Use "I" Statements**: Say, "I feel upset when you cancel plans at the last minute because I value our time together," instead of "You are so unreliable and selfish!"
3. **Listen Fully**: Let the other person finish explaining their point of view. Then summarize what they said to confirm you understand.
4. **Look for Solutions Together**: Ask, "How can we prevent this issue from happening again?" or "What do we both need to feel comfortable?"
5. **Know When to Pause**: If emotions run too high, take a short break to cool down. Return to the discussion with a clearer mind.

## Encouraging Growth in Others

Supportive relationships are not just about receiving help but also about giving it. Encourage your loved ones to pursue their dreams, learn new skills, and embrace positive changes.

- **Offer Specific Praise**: Instead of saying, "You're so great," try, "I'm really impressed by how you handled that customer's complaint at work." Specific compliments show you notice their efforts.
- **Ask About Goals**: Show genuine curiosity about what they hope to achieve, and ask how you can support them. Maybe that means offering to proofread a resume or watch their child for an hour so they can practice a skill.
- **Be an Accountability Partner**: If someone wants to start exercising, offer to do it together or check in weekly to see how they are doing.
- **Celebrate Milestones**: Did your friend complete a training course? Finish a big project? Let them know you see their success and are proud.

When you invest in others' growth, you strengthen the bond by showing you truly care about their well-being.

## Knowing When to Let Go

Sometimes, you can do everything right—communicate clearly, be empathetic, respect boundaries—but a relationship remains unhealthy. Maybe the other person dismisses your feelings or continues harmful behavior despite repeated discussions. In such cases, it might be time to step back or end the relationship entirely.

Letting go is rarely easy, especially if it involves a longtime friend or family member. It can feel painful or guilty. However, preserving your mental and emotional health is important. If a relationship constantly drains you, causes harm, or violates your sense of safety and self-respect, detachment might be the best path. That does not mean you wish the other person ill; it simply means you recognize the relationship no longer contributes positively to either of you.

## Technology's Role in Relationships

In today's world, technology can both help and hinder relationships. On the one hand, social media and messaging apps make it easier to stay in touch with people far away. On the other hand, relying solely on digital connections can lead to superficial interactions if we are not careful.

- **Stay Mindful of Screen Time**: If you spend more time scrolling through feeds than having real conversations, you might feel disconnected.
- **Use Technology Purposefully**: Video calls with distant loved ones or thoughtful text messages can maintain closeness. Just be sure to set aside time for face-to-face meetings if possible.
- **Avoid Misunderstandings**: Tone does not always come across in text, so be careful when discussing serious topics online. Sometimes a phone call or in-person chat is better.

## Personal Growth Through Relationships

Every person you meet has something to teach you—about the world, about yourself, or about how to relate to others. By viewing your relationships as opportunities to learn and grow, you maintain a sense of curiosity and humility. Ask yourself:

- What positive qualities does this person bring out in me?
- What challenges do they present that help me become more patient, understanding, or assertive?
- How can I apply lessons from our bond to other areas of my life?

This reflective approach turns even difficult interactions into learning experiences. While supportive relationships are certainly the easiest to embrace, complicated ones can also lead to personal insight if managed carefully.

# Chapter 12: Self-Care and Relaxation

## Introduction

With life's many demands—work, family, friendships, and personal goals—it is easy to forget one crucial relationship: the one you have with yourself. Self-care is about nurturing your physical, emotional, and mental well-being so you can handle challenges with a steady mind and maintain a healthy balance. Relaxation is a key part of self-care, yet many people treat it as a luxury or something that has to be earned. In reality, regular relaxation is essential for overall wellness.

This chapter will guide you through the importance of self-care, various relaxation techniques, and practical ways to incorporate restful moments into your day-to-day routine. By the end, you will see self-care not as an afterthought but as an integral part of who you are and how you live.

## Understanding Self-Care

Self-care covers a wide range of actions aimed at protecting and improving your well-being. It can be as simple as drinking enough water or as profound as seeking therapy to process deep emotional wounds. The core idea is that you deserve attention and care—just like the people you support or the tasks you handle.

Common myths about self-care include:

- **It is Selfish**: Actually, taking care of yourself helps you be more present and effective in helping others.
- **It Is Expensive**: While spa trips or fancy items can be part of self-care, so can free or low-cost activities like going for a walk, journaling, or listening to calming music.
- **It Takes Too Much Time**: Even short moments of self-care—like a five-minute breather at work—can make a difference.

When you practice consistent self-care, you are better able to manage stress, keep your relationships healthy, and stay focused on your personal growth.

## Identifying Your Self-Care Needs

Each person's self-care preferences differ based on their personality, lifestyle, and current life circumstances. What relaxes one person might bore another. Reflect on what truly helps you reset:

- **Physical Needs**: Do you need more sleep, a healthier diet, or regular exercise?
- **Emotional Needs**: Do you need quiet alone time, a good talk with a trusted friend, or creative outlets?
- **Mental Stimulation**: Do you feel energized by learning a new skill or reading a challenging book? Or do you prefer calming your mind with fewer inputs?

Take note of activities that leave you feeling refreshed rather than drained. If you are not sure, experiment. Try painting, yoga, cooking, or journaling, and see how you feel afterward.

## Incorporating Small Acts of Self-Care Daily

Many people skip self-care because they do not think they have time. However, small, consistent actions add up. Here are everyday ideas you can fit into any schedule:

1. **Mindful Breathing**: Pause for a minute or two to take slow, deep breaths. This can be done while waiting in line, riding the elevator, or during a break at work.
2. **Short Walks**: Even a quick stroll around the block can clear your head and get your blood moving.
3. **Hydration**: Keep a water bottle nearby. Make a habit of taking sips throughout the day.
4. **Positive Notes**: Jot down a quick positive affirmation or something you are grateful for. This shifts your mindset from stress to appreciation.
5. **Break from Screens**: Look away from electronic devices regularly. Blink, stretch your eyes, or gaze outside if you can.

These small pockets of self-care prevent you from reaching the end of the day feeling completely overwhelmed.

# Different Forms of Relaxation

Relaxation can take many forms—physical, mental, or emotional. The key is to find methods that genuinely soothe your body and mind.

**Physical Relaxation**

- **Progressive Muscle Relaxation**: Tense and release each muscle group from your toes to your head. This eases tension and trains you to notice when you are holding stress in your body.
- **Soothing Baths or Showers**: Warm water can relax tight muscles and calm your nervous system. You can enhance the experience with soft music or scented candles if you enjoy them.
- **Gentle Stretching or Yoga**: Focus on slow, controlled movements that help your body loosen up. Even simple stretches can release pent-up stress.

**Mental Relaxation**

- **Guided Imagery**: Close your eyes and picture a peaceful scene—perhaps a beach or a quiet forest. Imagine the colors, sounds, and scents in detail.
- **Meditation**: This practice can be as simple as focusing on your breathing or repeating a calming phrase. Some people use apps or online videos for guided sessions.
- **Reading or Listening to Music**: Immersing yourself in a good book or soothing music can shift your mind away from worries.

**Emotional Relaxation**

- **Journaling**: Writing out your thoughts and feelings can be cathartic, helping you process emotions and gain clarity.
- **Creative Activities**: Painting, crafting, or playing an instrument allows you to express feelings that words might not capture.
- **Talking to a Supportive Friend**: Sometimes the most relieving action is sharing your burdens with someone who listens without judgment.

## Setting Boundaries Around Rest

Just as we discussed setting boundaries in relationships (Chapter 6), you also need boundaries to protect your rest and relaxation time. This might mean saying "no" to extra tasks when you are already overloaded or turning off your phone at a certain hour every night. If you never defend the time you need to recharge, it will easily be taken up by other demands.

- **Create a Relaxation Schedule**: Decide on at least one chunk of time each day to relax, even if it is just 15 minutes.
- **Communicate Needs**: Let friends or family know when you are taking a break and prefer not to be disturbed, if possible.
- **Limit Interruptions**: Turn off unnecessary notifications or put your phone on "do not disturb" mode while you rest.

Even if you cannot fully disconnect from responsibilities (like if you are a parent of small children), you can still carve out small, consistent rest times. Making rest a priority prevents burnout and maintains emotional balance.

## Addressing Guilt About Taking Breaks

Many people, especially women, feel guilty about resting. You might think, "I should be doing something productive." However, rest is productive in its own way—by replenishing energy, boosting creativity, and reducing stress. If guilt arises, remind yourself:

1. **Health is Essential**: Without caring for yourself, you cannot be at your best for others.
2. **You Deserve It**: Everyone deserves downtime, no matter how busy life is.
3. **Balance Improves Productivity**: Studies show that short breaks actually lead to better focus and performance in the long run.

Over time, you can train your mind to view relaxation as a normal, necessary part of life, rather than a luxury you cannot afford.

## Creating a Relaxing Environment

Your surroundings can greatly impact your stress levels. Clutter, harsh lighting, or constant noise can all make relaxation difficult. Consider small adjustments:

- **Declutter Regularly**: A messy room can keep your mind uneasy. Clear out items you no longer need, and organize spaces so they are easy to maintain.
- **Soothing Colors and Lighting**: Soft lamps or natural light can create a calming atmosphere. If you can, add a plant or two for a touch of nature.
- **Comfortable Textures**: Cozy blankets, supportive pillows, or a soft rug can make a space more inviting.
- **Fresh Air**: If possible, open windows or use air purifiers to keep the air clean and refreshing.

These changes do not have to be expensive. Even rearranging furniture or adding a small candle can transform a room into a more peaceful retreat.

## Aligning Self-Care with Personal Values

In Chapter 9, we covered personal values. Aligning your self-care activities with those values can make them more meaningful. For instance, if you value creativity, painting or writing poetry might be especially rewarding. If you value connection, a weekly walk with a friend or a family member might help you relax.

Consider weaving your self-care into causes or passions you believe in. If you love nature, schedule time for a walk in the park or a picnic in a scenic area. If you value community service, volunteer at a local shelter or charity—just ensure this does not become another stressful obligation. The idea is to engage in activities that fill your heart with purpose as well as calm.

## Overcoming Common Self-Care Obstacles

Despite good intentions, everyday life can derail self-care plans. Here are some common obstacles and how to tackle them:

1. **Lack of Time**: Try micro self-care—quick but purposeful breaks throughout the day. Also, delegate tasks where possible or ask for help.
2. **Financial Constraints**: Remember that many relaxation methods are free or low-cost, such as breathing exercises, journaling, or simple at-home spa sessions.
3. **Family Obligations**: Communicate with family members about your need for a brief break. Even if you have children, consider a child swap with another parent so each of you gets personal time occasionally.

4. **Work Demands**: Schedule breaks in your calendar just as you would meetings. If you can, step away from your desk to have lunch or do some stretching.
5. **Internal Resistance**: Sometimes, you might not feel worthy of rest. Challenge this thought by reminding yourself that a rested mind and body handle work and relationships more effectively.

## Incorporating Mindfulness

Mindfulness is the practice of being fully present in the moment, without judgment. While it overlaps with meditation, it can be integrated into almost any activity:

- **Mindful Eating**: Instead of rushing through your meal, notice the flavors, textures, and smells. Put away your phone or other distractions.
- **Mindful Walking**: Pay attention to the rhythm of your steps and the scenery around you. Feel the air on your skin.
- **Mindful Chores**: Even washing dishes can be a moment of relaxation if you focus on the warmth of the water and the satisfaction of a clean plate.

This approach transforms mundane tasks into opportunities for calm, which is especially helpful when time is tight.

## Combining Self-Care with Exercise

Physical movement is not only good for the body, but it can also boost mental well-being. However, you do not need intense workouts to benefit. Consider gentler forms of exercise if you are looking for relaxation:

- **Yoga**: Combines poses with breath control, promoting balance, flexibility, and calm.
- **Pilates**: Focuses on core strength and controlled movements, often leading to reduced stress.
- **Tai Chi**: A slow, flowing martial art that fosters both mental clarity and physical harmony.
- **Leisurely Walks**: Being in nature, if possible, adds an extra layer of relaxation.

Exercise produces endorphins—chemicals in your brain that make you feel good. This can help combat stress or low moods.

## Using Technology Wisely

Technology can either help or hinder your self-care and relaxation efforts. Consider a balanced approach:

- **Helpful Tools**: Apps that offer guided meditation, relaxation music, or sleep stories can be part of a healthy routine.
- **Monitoring Screen Time**: If you find yourself scrolling late into the night, set a cutoff time to protect your sleep.
- **Digital Declutter**: Unsubscribe from unnecessary email lists and unfollow accounts that do not bring you joy or useful information.

Sometimes, going offline is the best way to recharge. Try scheduling "no-tech" periods, like an hour in the morning or a weekend day when you intentionally unplug.

## Long-Term Benefits of Self-Care and Relaxation

Regular self-care is not just about feeling momentary relief—though that is certainly beneficial. Over time, you may notice:

- **Better Stress Management**: You bounce back from challenges more easily.
- **Improved Health**: Lower stress levels can lead to better sleep and reduced risk of certain health issues.
- **Greater Emotional Stability**: You are less likely to snap at loved ones or become overwhelmed by minor setbacks.
- **Increased Productivity**: A rested mind is more focused and creative.
- **Enhanced Self-Worth**: You demonstrate to yourself that you are deserving of care and attention.

These benefits make self-care a crucial investment in your future, affecting everything from your career performance to your relationships.

## Adjusting Your Approach Over Time

Your self-care needs might change as your life circumstances evolve. A new job, a move, or becoming a parent can all demand new strategies. Be flexible and adapt your routine as needed. If an old method no longer works or bores you, try a new one. The key is to stay tuned in to your body and mind, recognizing when you feel tense, anxious, or drained, and responding with kindness and proactive care.

# Chapter 13: Balancing Family, Friends, and Personal Space

## Introduction

As you progress on your self-improvement journey, a key challenge often emerges: finding the right balance between family responsibilities, friendships, and the essential need for personal space. Many of us feel pulled in multiple directions—perhaps you have aging parents who need more help, children who require constant attention, friends expecting you to socialize regularly, and a career to manage on top of all that. On some days, it might feel impossible to juggle all these roles without losing your sense of self.

This chapter addresses the art of creating harmony in your relationships with family, friends, and your own private world. Striking this balance is not about giving less love or attention to those who matter; it is about learning how to allocate your time and energy so you can show up fully—both for yourself and for others. By the end, you will have a clearer idea of how to protect personal space while still nurturing close relationships.

---

## The Importance of Personal Space

Personal space is more than just physical distance. It also includes mental and emotional boundaries that help you maintain a sense of individuality and well-being. Without moments of solitude or self-reflection, you can become overwhelmed, easily irritated, or disconnected from your inner voice.

Yet, society often rewards people (especially women) for being available at all times—whether for family, friends, or work. This can lead to guilt when you try to carve out time for yourself. Recognizing personal space as a valid need is the first step. It is not selfish to say, "I need a moment to myself." It is an essential component of healthy living.

## Balancing Family Obligations

Family relationships usually top the list of priorities, especially if you are a parent, a caregiver, or a person who feels a strong sense of duty toward family members. While family bonds can be a source of incredible love and support, they can also become demanding if not managed carefully.

**Setting Family Expectations**

You may live with people who rely on you—children, a spouse, or other relatives. If they are used to having constant access to your time, it might come as a surprise when you start asserting your need for personal space or certain boundaries. The key is clear, compassionate communication. Explain that you love them and will still be there for them, but you also need quiet periods or alone time to recharge.

For example, if you have young children, you might schedule a "quiet hour" during the day when they read or play quietly in their rooms. If you live with a partner who wants to spend every evening together, propose a routine that includes a couple of nights for shared activities and one or two nights for independent downtime. These small shifts teach family members that your personal space is a normal and healthy part of daily life.

**Delegating and Sharing Responsibilities**

One major reason women struggle to find personal space is feeling solely responsible for household tasks. This can include cleaning, grocery shopping, cooking, helping kids with homework, or caring for elderly relatives. If you carry the entire load, you are less likely to have time for yourself.

Whenever possible, delegate or share responsibilities. Kids can often take on age-appropriate chores, and partners or siblings can learn new tasks to lighten the burden on you. This not only frees up more personal time but also empowers family members to develop useful life skills. Delegating is not an act of abandoning your responsibilities; it is about ensuring that the household functions as a team effort.

**Caring for Aging Parents**

If you have aging parents, you may feel a strong sense of responsibility to look after them. This is admirable, but it can also be emotionally demanding. Caregiving can expand to fill every spare moment if you do not set boundaries. See if siblings, other relatives, or even professional services (home care aides, adult day programs) can share the workload. Using resources like senior centers or respite care helps you maintain balance without neglecting your loved ones.

When you do spend time with aging parents, try to focus on quality over quantity. Make your visits meaningful—engage in real conversations, ask about their memories, or share small joys. This approach allows you to care for them with love while still preserving some personal space in your schedule.

---

## Nurturing Friendships

Friends offer laughter, companionship, and an outlet for sharing hopes and fears outside the family context. Yet friendships also demand time and emotional energy. Balancing multiple friendships with family obligations and personal needs can feel tricky.

**Quality Over Quantity**

Do you find yourself with a long list of acquaintances but only a few close friends? There is nothing wrong with having many casual contacts, but deeper friendships often require consistent effort. Instead of spreading yourself too thin, consider focusing on the relationships that truly enrich your life.

Ask yourself: Which friends lift you up and encourage your growth? Who respects your boundaries? In some cases, you may have outgrown certain friendships that once served you but now drain you. It is okay to let those fade if you find you are constantly exhausted or anxious after spending time with them.

**Setting Boundaries with Friends**

Friends can be wonderful, but sometimes they can also overstep. Perhaps you have a friend who calls at odd hours or expects immediate responses to texts. Or maybe a friend constantly unloads personal drama and rarely asks how you are doing. While it is good to be empathetic, you have a right to your own space.

Learn to assert your boundaries kindly. For instance, you can say, "I appreciate that you want to talk, but I'm not able to chat late at night anymore," or "I can meet for coffee on weekends, but I need weekday evenings free for family." True friends will understand. If they react negatively or accuse you of not caring, consider whether that friendship is truly respectful of your needs.

**Making Time for Friends Despite Busy Schedules**

When life gets hectic, friendships can be one of the first things to slip. Months may pass without a real conversation or meeting. While occasional breaks happen, investing in friendships can bring substantial emotional benefits.

- **Combine Social Time with Other Activities**: If you need to exercise, invite a friend for a walk instead of meeting at a restaurant. Or plan a cooking night if both of you enjoy trying new recipes. This way, you maintain your routine and catch up simultaneously.
- **Plan in Advance**: Busy schedules often require a bit of structure. If you know you are free on a certain weekend, schedule a friend get-together in advance so it is in both your calendars.
- **Stay Flexible**: If a friend cancels at the last minute, be understanding. Everyone faces demands on their time. Try to reschedule without drama, and they might be more understanding when you have to bow out as well.

---

## Protecting Your Personal Space

You may have already read about setting healthy boundaries in Chapter 6, but here, the focus is specifically on carving out physical and emotional space for yourself when you have a life brimming with relationships.

**Creating a Personal Retreat at Home**

If you share your living space with family or roommates, it might feel like there is nowhere to go for peace and quiet. However, even a small corner of your home can serve as a personal retreat if you claim it. This could be a comfortable chair by a window, a desk in a cozy corner, or even part of a closet that you transform into a "mini hideaway."

Decorate this area with items that calm you—soft lighting, a small plant, or personal mementos. If your space is limited, consider using headphones for soothing music or ambient sounds. If possible, establish a house rule that certain times of the day or week are for you to be alone in this space, uninterrupted.

**Scheduling Solitude**

One effective tactic is treating personal time like any other appointment. Block it out on your calendar. It could be 30 minutes in the morning before others wake up, an hour in the evening after dinner, or a specific weekend afternoon. Label it as "Me Time" or "Personal Space" and do your best not to compromise on it unless there is an emergency.

Using this scheduled solitude intentionally matters. It is not just about scrolling on social media or watching random videos—though some light entertainment can be part of it. Try journaling, meditating, reading, or simply sitting quietly. Let your mind wander and decompress from the constant noise of daily obligations.

**Handling Guilt**

Feeling guilty about taking personal time is common. You might think, "I should be helping with homework" or "I should be calling my friend back." But remember, maintaining personal space allows you to show up more fully when you do engage with family or friends. If you constantly run on empty, your relationships will suffer in the long run.

Challenge negative self-talk by affirming that rest and personal space are valid needs. Keep reminding yourself that by recharging, you can be more patient, more loving, and more supportive to the people who need you.

---

## Managing Overlapping Social Circles

For many adults, family members become friends, or vice versa, which can blur lines. You might have a cousin who is also your best friend, or a friend who practically lives with you like family. While this closeness can be wonderful, it also means you have fewer clear boundaries between different parts of your life.

Define roles and expectations carefully. For instance, if you have a cousin who visits frequently and treats your home like a second house, talk about any guidelines or schedules you need. Make sure your personal space remains respected. On the flip side, if you enjoy this overlapping connection, decide on shared routines that bring a sense of stability—like planning a big family-friend dinner once a week but leaving other evenings free.

---

## Handling Special Situations

Sometimes, life events create special circumstances that demand more time and energy. Examples include:

- **New Parent**: Balancing a newborn's needs with time for your partner, other children, and yourself can be overwhelming. You might need to rely on extended family or close friends to step in occasionally so you can rest or refocus.
- **Serious Illness in the Family**: If a relative is sick, you may suddenly have to juggle hospital visits, medical paperwork, and emotional support. During these times, do not neglect your own health. Lean on friends for meal support or babysitting, and remember that your own well-being matters.
- **Major Career Shift**: Taking on a new job or launching a business might temporarily shift your priorities. Inform your family and friends that your schedule is changing. Ask for patience, but also plan short check-ins so you do not vanish entirely from your social world.

In all these cases, communication is crucial. Let your loved ones know what is happening, what kind of help you need, and when you might need more personal space to cope. Most people want to be supportive if you give them clear guidelines.

---

## The Art of Saying "No" Gracefully

One significant aspect of balance is learning to say "no." You might feel obligated to attend every birthday party, volunteer for every school event, or accept every social invitation from friends. Yet, spreading yourself too thin can lead to stress, resentment, or burnout.

Saying "no" does not mean rejecting the person; it is about declining the request. A simple "I'm sorry, I can't make it this time" or "I wish I could help, but my schedule is full right now" is enough. You do not need to give detailed explanations or excuses unless you want to. Being direct but polite helps others understand and usually prevents hurt feelings. Often, people will respect you more for knowing and honoring your limits.

---

## When Relationships Become Unbalanced

Sometimes, family or friends may continually take from you—your time, your emotional energy—without offering the same level of support in return. While relationships should not be calculated on a 50/50 scale every day, chronic imbalance can be draining. If you feel you are always the giver and rarely the receiver, it might be time for a candid conversation.

Ask yourself some questions:

- **Have I clearly voiced my needs, or am I expecting them to guess?**
- **Is this person capable of giving more, or are they in a season of life where they genuinely cannot?**
- **Do I need to adjust my expectations or step back?**

Sometimes, setting new boundaries or lowering your emotional investment can restore balance. In other cases, you might realize the relationship is not healthy for you in its current form. While letting go is difficult (as mentioned in Chapter 11), it can be necessary to protect your mental and emotional space.

---

## Respecting Others' Space

Balance goes both ways. Just as you need your own personal space, others need theirs. If a friend or family member asks for some alone time, try not to take it personally. Everyone has different limits for social interaction. Respecting these differences is part of building stable, trusting relationships.

If a loved one seems withdrawn or stressed, consider gently asking if they need more room to decompress. Encouraging them to speak openly about their boundaries can strengthen your bond because you demonstrate genuine care for their well-being.

---

## Strategies for Sustaining Balance

Maintaining balance among family, friends, and personal space is not a one-time action; it is an ongoing process. Life changes, schedules shift, and relationships evolve. Here are some overarching strategies:

1. **Regular Check-Ins**: Periodically review how you feel. Are you overwhelmed? Are you missing alone time? Are certain relationships draining you? Awareness is key to making timely adjustments.
2. **Shared Calendars**: If you share a household, a family calendar (physical or digital) can make scheduling easier. It reduces conflicts by making everyone aware of each other's commitments and rest times.
3. **Self-Care Rituals**: Keep practicing self-care and relaxation (Chapter 12). When you invest in your own well-being, you have more energy to navigate family and social life.
4. **Flexibility with Structure**: Having some structure is good—set meal times, planned outings, scheduled personal time—but stay flexible. Unexpected events will happen, and you may need to adapt. Just ensure you find a new balance afterward.
5. **Ask for Help**: Whether it is child care, a shoulder to cry on, or advice about a tough family situation, do not hesitate to reach out to your network. You do not have to manage everything by yourself.

# Chapter 14: Creativity and Self-Discovery

## Introduction

Creativity is not limited to painting a masterpiece or writing a novel. It is an open door to exploring ideas, expressing emotions, and finding hidden parts of yourself. When you tap into your creative energy—whether through art, music, problem-solving, or simply daydreaming—you often unlock deeper layers of self-discovery. This chapter looks at how creativity can be a powerful tool in your ongoing journey toward personal growth.

You might think, "I'm not creative" or "I can't draw or sing." But creativity is not a skill reserved for professional artists. It lives in everyday activities: writing in a journal, rearranging furniture, cooking a new recipe, or brainstorming solutions at work. As you dive in, you might be surprised at the insights you gain about yourself—your tastes, your passions, and even your untapped potential.

---

## Defining Creativity

Creativity often involves producing something original or thinking of a new approach to a familiar topic. It can also be a process of self-expression that lets you capture emotions or experiences in a unique format. The goal is not always a final product; sometimes, the act of creating is where the magic lies.

Examples of creative expressions include:

- Making music or playing an instrument.
- Sculpting, painting, sketching, or doodling.
- Writing stories, poetry, or personal reflections.
- Designing a home or garden space.
- Inventing new recipes or experimenting with flavors.
- Approaching everyday tasks (like problem-solving at work) with fresh thinking.

Any time you generate ideas and shape them into something tangible—whether physical or conceptual—you are exercising your creative muscles. Creativity can be playful, serious, or anywhere in between.

---

## How Creativity Fuels Self-Discovery

When you engage in creative pursuits, you become more in tune with your thoughts and feelings. For example, writing a short story can reveal personal themes or experiences you did not realize were significant. Painting an abstract picture might help you release pent-up emotions. Solving a complicated puzzle could highlight your resilience and problem-solving style.

Creativity is a gateway to self-discovery because it often bypasses the logical filters that tell you what you "should" think or feel. Instead, you can explore freely, letting your intuition guide you. In this process, you might notice patterns—like always leaning toward bright colors or certain story themes—that indicate unspoken desires or deep-seated values. These insights can inform other areas of your life, such as career choices, relationship preferences, or personal goals.

---

## Overcoming Creative Blocks

Many people avoid creative activities because they fear they are "not good enough." However, the true value of creativity lies in the journey, not external approval. If you feel stuck or intimidated, consider these approaches:

1. **Freewriting**: Set a timer for 10 minutes and write without stopping or editing. Let your thoughts flow, even if they seem random or silly. This helps silence your inner critic.
2. **Doodling or Scribbling**: Keep a small notebook for doodles. Draw whatever comes to mind without worrying about technique or style.
3. **Creative Prompts**: Use prompts from books, websites, or apps. For instance, a writing prompt might ask you to describe a day in the life of an inanimate object. A drawing prompt might suggest "illustrate your favorite dream."

4. **Collaborations**: Sometimes working with someone else can spark creativity. You can bounce ideas off each other or take turns adding to a shared project.
5. **Embrace Mistakes**: Accept that creativity is messy. A failed attempt often teaches you more than an easy success. Laugh off the results that do not match your expectations and keep going.

---

## Finding Your Preferred Medium

Not every creative outlet will resonate with you. Some people love journaling but dislike painting. Others find dance or photography more engaging. Experiment with different forms until you discover what feels natural and exciting.

- **Visual Arts**: Painting, drawing, collage, or even coloring books if you want a more guided experience.
- **Performing Arts**: Singing, dancing, acting, or playing an instrument.
- **Literary Arts**: Creative writing, poetry, journaling, or blogging.
- **Crafts and DIY**: Knitting, sewing, woodworking, or upcycling old items.
- **Digital Creations**: Graphic design, video editing, digital art, or coding for fun projects.
- **Everyday Creativity**: Decorating your home, cooking, gardening, or organizing events with a creative touch.

Your chosen medium can be private—like a secret diary—or public, like performing on a stage. Both approaches have value. The important part is that you genuinely enjoy the process or find meaning in it.

---

## The Role of Curiosity

Curiosity sparks creativity. When you are curious, you ask questions like, "What if…?" or "How could I…?" This mindset opens up possibilities. For instance, if you are curious about a new recipe, you might experiment with ingredients you have never tried before. If you are curious about a social issue, you might craft a poem or painting that expresses your viewpoint.

You can nurture curiosity by observing the world around you. Take walks without headphones, noticing sights, sounds, and smells. Read articles or watch documentaries outside your usual interests. Chat with people who have different life experiences. Each time you learn something new or spot something intriguing, your creative brain gets fresh material to work with.

## Connecting Creativity to Emotional Healing

Creativity can also play a therapeutic role, helping you cope with emotional pain, anxiety, or past traumas. This does not replace professional therapy, but it can complement it. Writing a letter to your younger self or painting a scene that represents a painful memory can provide a sense of release and understanding. Some people find that artistic expression helps them articulate feelings they struggle to put into words.

If you are dealing with overwhelming emotions, consider art journaling—a method where you combine writing with drawing, collage, or painting in a single journal. You can create pages for your hopes, fears, or memories. Over time, seeing how your journal evolves can be both healing and empowering.

## Building Confidence Through Creativity

Each time you finish a creative project—no matter how small—you give yourself proof that you can start and complete something. This fosters a sense of capability. Even if you do not show your work to anyone, knowing you made it can boost self-esteem.

Moreover, creativity often involves risk-taking. You might try a new technique or reveal something personal. When you succeed or learn from the attempt, you realize you are more resilient than you thought. This self-assuredness can spill into other areas of life. For instance, you might feel bolder about sharing ideas at work or initiating new social connections, knowing you are capable of handling uncertainty.

## Incorporating Creativity Into Daily Life

You do not need large blocks of time to benefit from creative activities. Even a few minutes can be refreshing. Here are ways to sprinkle creativity into your routines:

- **Morning Pages**: Write three pages of stream-of-consciousness thoughts right after you wake up. This method, popularized by Julia Cameron in "The Artist's Way," helps clear mental clutter and ignite creativity.
- **Spontaneous Sketches**: Keep a small sketchpad in your bag. When you have a spare moment—on public transit or during a lunch break—sketch your surroundings.
- **Cooking Experiments**: Instead of always following recipes, try improvising a dish with what you have in the fridge. Notice flavors and textures, adjusting as you go.
- **Mini Creative Challenges**: Challenge yourself to craft one haiku a day, snap one interesting photo, or write a four-line poem before bedtime.

By making creativity a consistent habit, you gradually open yourself to new insights and self-discovery without feeling overwhelmed or pressured to produce perfect work.

---

## Overcoming Perfectionism

One common creativity blocker is perfectionism—the idea that every piece of art or writing must be flawless. This mind-set can stifle experimentation. Remember, creativity thrives on trial, error, and happy accidents. If you find yourself hesitating to start a project because you fear it will not be "good," try these strategies:

- **Set a "Bad First Draft" Goal**: Aim to create something unpolished on purpose. Tell yourself, "I'm just going to create a rough, imperfect version." Once the pressure to be perfect is gone, you free up the flow of ideas.
- **Create for Your Eyes Only**: Sometimes you just need to keep your work private, so you do not worry about external judgment. After finishing, you can decide if you want to share it or not.

- **Celebrate Imperfections**: If a painting or poem does not turn out as planned, look for parts you do like. Maybe the color choices were interesting, or a particular phrase resonates. Let that be your focus instead of obsessing over flaws.

Learning to let go of perfection allows you to fully immerse yourself in the creative experience, which is the real treasure.

---

## Collaborating and Sharing Your Creations

While private creativity can be immensely rewarding, sharing or collaborating with others can add another layer of growth. Presenting your work in a safe, supportive environment—like a writing group or local art club—can boost your confidence and help you receive constructive feedback. Just be sure the group's atmosphere is genuinely encouraging, not overly critical or elitist.

Collaboration, such as co-writing a short story or co-creating a painting, can spark fresh ideas and teach you how to merge different visions. It also hones your communication skills as you learn to negotiate creative differences. Whether the final result is showcased publicly or just shared among friends, the process itself can be enlightening.

---

## Linking Creativity to Other Personal Growth Areas

Creativity ties neatly to many themes explored in earlier chapters:

- **Stress Management (Chapters 7 & 8)**: Engaging in a craft or art can serve as a form of relaxation. Painting, writing, or playing music can lower anxiety by absorbing you in the present moment.
- **Values and Purpose (Chapter 9)**: If you value empathy, you might use your art to highlight social issues. If adventure is a core value, you might experiment with bold mediums or content that challenges your comfort zone.
- **Career Growth (Chapter 10)**: Creative thinking can help you solve work problems more innovatively. It might also lead you to explore career

paths in design, communication, or project development that align with your new interests.
- **Relationships (Chapters 11 & 13)**: You can collaborate on creative projects with family or friends, strengthening bonds. Alternatively, having a creative hobby offers you a personal outlet that balances the demands of relationships.

Seeing creativity as interconnected rather than an isolated activity makes it easier to keep it central in your life.

---

## Staying Motivated on the Creative Path

Just like with any pursuit, there can be ebbs and flows in creative energy. Some days you will be eager to paint or write; other days, you might feel uninspired.

- **Create a Ritual**: Light a candle, put on certain music, or sip a favorite tea whenever you begin your creative work. The brain often responds to ritual by switching into a focused mode.
- **Join a Challenge**: Many online communities host monthly or weekly creative challenges—like "Inktober" for drawing or "NaNoWriMo" for novel writing. These can push you to keep creating regularly.
- **Limit Distractions**: Turn off notifications or find a quiet space. If you only have 20 minutes, make those 20 minutes count by giving your full attention to the project.
- **Reflect on Your Why**: Remind yourself why creativity matters to you—perhaps it helps you relax, discover new sides of yourself, or connect with others on a deeper level.

If you hit a creative slump, try something new: a different medium, a new prompt, or a fresh environment. Keep experimenting, and do not be afraid to step back for a short break if you feel utterly stuck. Sometimes distance can reignite inspiration.

## Embracing Growth and Change

As you continue exploring creativity, you may notice you are drawn to different styles or themes over time. What excited you last month may not excite you next year—and that is okay. Let your interests evolve. Each stage of creative exploration reflects your growth as a person.

You might develop a particular style or voice that people recognize as yours, or you could remain a creative chameleon who experiments constantly. Neither approach is superior. The real aim is self-discovery and expression, which can look different for each individual.

---

## Practical Exercises for Creative Self-Discovery

1. **Dream Board or Vision Collage**: Gather images, words, and colors that appeal to you from magazines or printouts. Paste them on a poster to represent your hopes and dreams, even if they seem random. See what patterns emerge.
2. **Character Sketches**: If you like writing, invent characters and write short paragraphs describing their personalities or backgrounds. Notice any elements that reflect parts of yourself.
3. **Musical Journaling**: Make a short playlist each week that captures your current mood. Jot down why you chose each song. This helps you track emotional changes and discover what music resonates with you.
4. **Color Emotions**: Assign a color to each emotion you experience throughout the day. At night, paint or sketch blocks of color in proportion to how much of each emotion you felt. Over time, see if certain colors dominate.
5. **Random Inspiration**: Flip to a random page in a dictionary or encyclopedia. Whatever word or concept you land on, create something related to it—a quick poem, a doodle, or a short essay. This breaks routine thinking and sparks novelty.

These activities are playful yet revealing, offering new angles on your inner world. They are not about producing a masterpiece; they are about learning, healing, and celebrating who you are.

# Chapter 15: Positive Thinking and Growth Mindset

## Introduction

Life is full of ups and downs. While you cannot always control external events, you can shape how you respond to them. That is where positive thinking and a growth mindset come in. Positive thinking involves focusing on constructive possibilities rather than dwelling on negativity. A growth mindset is the belief that you can learn, improve, and adapt through effort and experience—even when you face challenges. Together, they can help you overcome obstacles, maintain resilience, and foster an attitude of continuous self-improvement.

In this chapter, we will explore what it means to embrace a more optimistic outlook on life, the difference between fixed and growth mindsets, and practical ways to train your mind to stay open and hopeful even in tough situations. By the end, you will understand why cultivating positive thinking and a growth mindset does not mean ignoring reality—but rather, choosing to see possibilities where others see only limitations.

---

## Understanding Positive Thinking

**Positive thinking** is not about pretending everything is perfect. Instead, it means acknowledging problems without losing sight of potential solutions or the lessons a situation might offer. It is about giving your focus to what can be done rather than what cannot be changed.

### Benefits of Positive Thinking

1. **Reduced Stress**: When you approach life with optimism, stressors may still occur, but you are less likely to spiral into panic or despair.
2. **Better Emotional Health**: Constructive thought patterns can lead to fewer episodes of anxiety, anger, or hopelessness.
3. **Improved Problem-Solving**: People who believe solutions exist often spot them faster.

4. **Enhanced Relationships**: An optimistic demeanor can positively influence those around you, improving teamwork and cooperation.

Positive thinking does not eliminate problems. It helps you face them with clearer eyes and a calmer spirit, which often leads to more effective actions.

---

## Recognizing Negative Thought Patterns

Everyone has negative thoughts sometimes. But if they dominate your mind, they can distort your view of what is possible. Common negative patterns include:

- **Catastrophizing**: Immediately assuming the worst-case scenario.
- **Overgeneralizing**: Using one event to define all others, like thinking "I messed up this project, so I'm a failure at everything."
- **All-or-Nothing Thinking**: Viewing things in extremes, with no gray area—for example, "I must be perfect, or I'm a total loser."
- **Mind Reading**: Concluding you know what others think (usually something bad) without real evidence.

When you notice these patterns, pause and question them. Are they based on facts, or on fear and assumption? Challenging negative thoughts helps you replace them with a more balanced perspective.

---

## Shifting Toward a Positive Mindset

Moving away from chronic pessimism or self-criticism takes time and practice. Here are a few methods:

1. **Thought Replacement**
   Each time you catch a negative thought, replace it with one that is more constructive or hopeful. For example, change "I'll never finish this on time" to "I can ask for help or rearrange my schedule to get this done."
2. **Positive Affirmations**
   Short, uplifting statements you repeat to yourself, such as, "I am capable

of learning and improving," or "I trust myself to find solutions." These can feel cheesy at first, but over time, they can rewire your habitual thinking.
3. **Focus on Small Wins**
Instead of waiting for huge successes, notice and celebrate small achievements—finishing a daily workout, completing a work task early, or even just having a pleasant conversation. Acknowledging tiny victories builds a sense of progress and encourages further optimism.
4. **Seek the Lesson**
When something goes wrong, ask, "What can I learn from this?" This question redirects your mind away from failure and toward growth.

---

## The Growth Mindset vs. Fixed Mindset

Psychologist Carol Dweck introduced the concept of **growth mindset** versus **fixed mindset**. A fixed mindset believes that abilities (intelligence, talent) are static traits—you either have them or you do not. A growth mindset sees abilities as skills you can develop over time.

**Key Differences**

- **Reaction to Failure**:
    - *Fixed Mindset*: Feels exposed—failure is proof of lack of ability.
    - *Growth Mindset*: Views failure as an opportunity to learn what went wrong and try again.
- **Response to Challenges**:
    - *Fixed Mindset*: May avoid challenges to protect the image of being "smart" or "talented."
    - *Growth Mindset*: Embraces challenges as a chance to get better.
- **Effort**:
    - *Fixed Mindset*: Believes needing effort is a sign of weakness or lack of talent.
    - *Growth Mindset*: Recognizes effort as a crucial part of improvement.

Cultivating a growth mindset can transform how you approach goals, relationships, and self-development. It opens doors to continuous learning and adaptability.

## Embracing Mistakes as Part of Learning

No one likes making mistakes, but they are inevitable when you step outside your comfort zone. A growth mindset reframes mistakes as data. Each error shows you what to adjust next time.

- **Identify Specific Lessons**: If you failed a test or messed up a presentation, figure out what specifically went wrong. Did you not study enough? Did you rush through your slides?
- **Adjust Your Strategy**: Use that insight to change your approach. This might mean studying longer, practicing your speech more thoroughly, or seeking feedback from someone knowledgeable.
- **Move On**: After you have learned what you can, let go of the guilt or embarrassment. Holding onto negative emotions about a past mistake stalls progress.

This approach is not about excusing errors; it is about growing from them. Over time, you will gain confidence in your ability to adapt, because you know you can handle setbacks constructively.

---

## Self-Compassion in the Growth Process

A key element of maintaining a positive outlook and growth mindset is treating yourself with compassion. When you scold yourself harshly for not mastering something immediately, you reinforce a fixed mindset (the idea that struggling means you are incapable). Instead, talk to yourself as you would to a friend in the same situation:

- **Acknowledge Feelings**: "I'm frustrated that I didn't do as well as I hoped."
- **Offer Reassurance**: "It's okay to feel disappointed. This does not mean I can't improve."
- **Encourage Action**: "Next time, I'll start practicing earlier or ask for extra help."

This balanced self-talk calms your mind and keeps you open to the learning process. It also prevents the paralyzing shame that can arise from repeated self-criticism.

## Building Optimism in Challenging Times

Positive thinking does not mean ignoring difficulties or injustice. However, it does mean choosing to see potential avenues for change. If you are going through a particularly rough phase—like job loss, relationship troubles, or health concerns—deliberately searching for positives can maintain your mental resilience.

- **Find Meaning**: Ask yourself how this challenge could lead to personal growth. Maybe losing your job pushes you to discover a new career path. Maybe health issues help you recognize what truly matters in life.
- **Practice Gratitude**: Even on hard days, try to find at least one thing you are thankful for—support from a friend, a comfortable bed, a moment of laughter. Gratitude shifts your focus to what you still have, rather than what is missing.
- **Stay Connected**: Isolation can deepen pessimism. Reach out to supportive friends, family, or professional counselors who can help you see the bigger picture and remind you of your strengths.

Over time, these habits train your brain to seek hope and solutions rather than giving in to despair.

---

## Surrounding Yourself with Positivity

Your environment can either boost or sabotage your attempts at positive thinking. Notice the kinds of people, media, and activities you allow into your life:

- **Supportive People**: Spend time with those who encourage you and challenge you to grow, rather than those who constantly complain or belittle your efforts.
- **Media Consumption**: News and social media can be overwhelming. While you cannot (and should not) ignore the world's problems, try balancing difficult news with inspirational stories or learning content that enriches your mind.
- **Positive Influences**: Listen to podcasts, read books, or watch videos that teach you something new or uplift your spirits. Interacting with positive material regularly reinforces your optimistic outlook.

You cannot always avoid negativity, but you can manage how frequently you expose yourself to it and how much weight you give it in your thoughts.

## Setting Realistic Goals

A growth mindset and positive thinking are most effective when paired with clear, achievable goals. If your targets are so high that you feel defeated before you begin, it can undermine your optimism. Break big ambitions into smaller milestones:

- **Short-Term Goals**: "I will complete this online course in 4 weeks."
- **Medium-Term Goals**: "I will apply the new skills from the course to improve my work performance within 3 months."
- **Long-Term Goals**: "I aim to transition into a more advanced role or a new field by next year."

Reaching smaller, short-term goals keeps your motivation high. Each success story becomes evidence that your effort and mindset lead to results, fueling even greater optimism for the next step.

## Visualizing Success (and Obstacles)

Another way to strengthen a growth mindset is **visualization**. This involves imagining yourself succeeding but also picturing potential obstacles:

1. **Envision Success**: Close your eyes and see yourself accomplishing your goal—finishing a race, delivering a speech, or getting that promotion. Notice how it feels.
2. **Anticipate Challenges**: Then, imagine the possible bumps along the way—an injury, fear of public speaking, extra competition for the promotion. This is not negativity but strategic thinking.
3. **Plan Responses**: Create mental action steps for how you will handle each obstacle. This prepares you psychologically and prevents panic if setbacks occur in real life.

Visualization helps align your mindset with both optimism and practical readiness. You remain hopeful about the outcome while acknowledging that difficulties can arise.

## Handling Doubts from Others

When you adopt a growth mindset and a positive outlook, not everyone will cheer you on. Some might scoff or accuse you of being unrealistic. Others may feel threatened if your optimism and can-do attitude highlight their own reluctance to change. How to respond?

- **Respect Different Views**: Recognize that not everyone is ready for a growth mindset. Changing perspectives takes personal readiness.
- **Explain Your Stance**: If someone is curious (rather than dismissive), share why you believe in continuous learning and positive thinking. Offer examples of how it has helped you solve problems or cope with stress.
- **Protect Your Energy**: If certain individuals constantly demean or mock your efforts, consider limiting your interactions with them. It is healthy to keep some distance from people who undermine your progress.

Remember, your journey is your own. While having encouragement is wonderful, you do not need universal approval to keep growing.

---

## Practical Exercises to Strengthen a Growth Mindset

1. **Daily Reflection**: Write down one challenge you faced each day and what you learned. Even if it is small, like a difficult conversation, note how you handled it and what you might do differently next time.
2. **Compliment Your Effort**: When you complete a task—big or small—acknowledge the effort you put in. "I did not give up even though it was tough," or "I spent extra time learning a skill, and it paid off."
3. **List of Growth Moments**: At the end of each week, list ways you improved, things you discovered, or fears you confronted. This helps you see that growth is ongoing, even if results are not immediate.
4. **Mentor or Role Model**: Identify a person who exemplifies a growth mindset—someone in your life, or a public figure. Reflect on how they respond to setbacks. Use their behavior as inspiration for how to handle your own challenges.

## Balancing Optimism with Realism

A positive outlook should never blind you to real dangers or issues. Overly naive thinking can lead to risky decisions because you might ignore warning signs. Aim for **optimistic realism**: you see the potential for success but also plan for potential setbacks. This approach keeps you hopeful while preventing careless mistakes.

- **Example**: If you want to start a small business, a purely "positive" approach might lead you to skip market research because you believe everything will work out. **Optimistic realism** means you do the research, plan for costs, and stay confident you can adapt if challenges arise.

This balance ensures your growth mindset remains grounded. You stay enthusiastic but also make informed choices.

---

## Sustaining a Growth Mindset Over Time

Like any habit, a growth mindset requires ongoing commitment. You might feel energetic at first but slip back into old thinking patterns under stress. Be patient with yourself, and remember that every moment of doubt is another chance to practice.

- **Continued Learning**: Keep reading, taking courses, or exploring new skills. The act of learning itself reinforces the idea that you can expand your abilities.
- **Periodic Goal Reviews**: Check in on your goals monthly or quarterly. Are you making progress? If not, is the goal too big, or do you need a new strategy?
- **Celebrate All Progress**: Growth mindset is about the journey. Even if you do not reach a milestone as fast as you hoped, celebrate the new knowledge or resilience you gained along the way.

Over time, you will see your perspective solidify. Challenges that once intimidated you may start to feel like natural steps toward growth.

# Chapter 16: Adapting to Change and Life Challenges

## Introduction

Change is a constant in life. People switch jobs, move to new cities, experience shifts in relationships, or face unforeseen crises like losing a loved one. Even positive events—like getting married or having a baby—can turn your routines upside down. Handling change effectively is essential for personal growth and emotional stability.

In this chapter, we will delve into why change can feel so intimidating, the different types of life challenges you might encounter, and practical strategies to stay grounded during transitions. By the end, you will see that adaptability is not just about surviving difficult times; it is about learning, evolving, and sometimes even finding unexpected opportunities in the midst of upheaval.

---

## Why Change Feels Unsettling

Human beings often crave a sense of security. Familiar routines, places, and people provide comfort because we know what to expect. When change disrupts this familiarity, it can trigger anxiety, fear, or resistance. Part of you might ask, "Will I be okay?" or "What if I can't handle this?" These questions are normal but can become overwhelming if left unchecked.

The good news is that humans are also incredibly adaptable. History is filled with stories of individuals who rebuilt their lives after major losses, or found success in a new field after being laid off. By recognizing that change—though uncomfortable—can also be a doorway to personal growth, you position yourself to adapt rather than be paralyzed by worry.

---

## Types of Life Challenges and Transitions

Change can manifest in many ways, each requiring a slightly different response:

1. **Career Changes**: Switching jobs, being laid off, or starting a new business can prompt excitement but also insecurity.
2. **Relationship Shifts**: Marriage, divorce, breakups, or evolving friendships. These events often affect living arrangements, finances, and emotional well-being.
3. **Health Crises**: A sudden illness, injury, or diagnosis can upend daily routines and priorities.
4. **Moving or Relocation**: Leaving a familiar community to live somewhere new involves practical logistics and emotional adjustment.
5. **Family Dynamics**: Births, adoptions, caring for elderly parents, or dealing with grief after losing a family member.
6. **Personal Growth Milestones**: Graduating from school, starting or ending a creative project, shifting life philosophies, or any major shift in self-perception.

The common thread among all these changes is that they alter your normal patterns. Awareness of the types of challenges you might face can help you prepare mentally before you are deep in the whirlwind.

---

## Emotional Responses to Change

When faced with a big transition, you might cycle through several emotions:

- **Denial**: Pretending the change is not real or is not significant.
- **Anger or Frustration**: Feeling resentful that you have to adjust.
- **Bargaining**: Hoping you can avoid the change by making certain compromises.
- **Sadness or Anxiety**: Mourning the loss of your old routine or fearing the unknown.
- **Acceptance**: Eventually coming to terms with the new reality.

These stages are similar to the stages of grief, though not everyone experiences them in a neat order. Recognizing these emotional phases can help you understand why you feel unsettled and reassure you that these feelings are part of the process.

## Strategies for Adapting to Change

Adapting does not mean you have to love the new situation right away, but it does mean finding ways to function and grow within it. Here are some approaches:

1. **Acknowledge Your Feelings**
   Let yourself feel sadness, frustration, or fear if it arises. Bottling up emotions can lead to more stress. Journaling, talking to a friend, or seeing a counselor can help you process these feelings.
2. **Stay Grounded in Self-Care**
   During transitions, routines often get disrupted—sleep schedules, eating habits, exercise. Try to maintain or re-establish simple self-care habits (see Chapter 12). Small acts like walking daily or doing short breathing exercises can anchor you when everything feels chaotic.
3. **Focus on What You Can Control**
   Certain aspects of change are outside your influence. Instead of wasting energy on the uncontrollable, direct your attention to what you can manage—like learning new skills, adjusting your schedule, or seeking help from supportive people.
4. **Break Down the Transition**
   Large changes can seem overwhelming. If you have moved to a new city, for example, tackle small tasks: explore your neighborhood, sign up for a local meetup, or find a primary care doctor. Each completed task builds confidence.
5. **Set Realistic Expectations**
   It takes time to adjust to a big shift. Do not expect to feel "at home" in a new job or city within days. Be patient with yourself, and acknowledge that adaptation is a process.

## Cultivating Flexibility

Being flexible means staying open to adjusting your plans as needed. If you are too rigid, you might miss better solutions or opportunities. For instance, if you lose your job, an inflexible mindset might cause you to only look for the same exact position. A flexible approach might let you consider adjacent roles or even an entirely new career path that suits your evolving interests.

**How to Practice Flexibility**:

- **Try New Experiences**: Even small acts, like trying a new cuisine or learning a different workout, train your brain to see variety as normal.
- **Embrace Feedback**: Whether from a boss, a friend, or your own reflections, feedback can guide you toward better approaches—if you stay open to it.
- **Let Go of "Should"**: Statements like, "I should be at this level by now" or "Things should be the way they used to be" cause stress. Instead, deal with what is actually happening, not what you feel you are owed.

This openness makes you more resilient because you are not trapped by a single way of thinking or doing.

---

## Harnessing a Growth Mindset for Transitions

From the previous chapter, you already know how a **growth mindset** supports learning and improvement. In the context of change:

- **See Challenges as Opportunities**: Ask, "How can this transition help me grow?" Instead of resisting a new situation, figure out what skills or insights you can gain.
- **Remain Curious**: Investigate your new environment or circumstances. Curiosity replaces dread with a sense of exploration.
- **Persist Through Setbacks**: If your first efforts to adapt fail, treat it as data. Adjust and try again. This iterative approach can make transitions smoother in the long run.

By merging adaptability with a growth mindset, you become better equipped to handle whatever life throws your way.

## Building a Support System

You do not have to face major changes alone. Leaning on others for help can speed your adjustment and provide emotional relief.

- **Friends and Family**: Share your feelings and experiences openly, even if you worry about seeming vulnerable. Trusted loved ones often want to help, but they cannot unless they know what you are going through.
- **Professional Help**: Therapists or coaches are trained to guide people through life's challenges. Seeking counseling is not a sign of weakness; it is a proactive step to ensure you have the tools to cope.
- **Community Resources**: Local groups or online forums can connect you with people who have faced similar changes, like support groups for new parents, those dealing with grief, or career-changers. Their experiences and advice can offer reassurance that you are not alone.

Be careful not to isolate yourself out of pride or fear. A strong support network can make all the difference in how quickly and gracefully you adapt.

## Financial Preparedness for Change

Many life challenges have a financial element. Planning for emergencies can reduce stress when unexpected expenses occur. Even small steps—like setting aside a portion of each paycheck into savings—build a cushion over time.

- **Emergency Fund**: Aim for at least three to six months' worth of living expenses saved if possible. This way, job loss or a sudden medical bill does not instantly plunge you into crisis.
- **Insurance Coverage**: Health, property, or life insurance can protect you in certain emergencies. Review your policies annually to ensure they still meet your needs.

- **Budget Adjustments**: If you anticipate a major change—like going back to school or taking unpaid leave—plan your finances well in advance. Cut unnecessary costs or find ways to earn extra income during transitional periods.

Being proactive about finances gives you one less thing to worry about when you are already dealing with big shifts in other areas of life.

## Coping with Uncertainty

Change often goes hand in hand with uncertainty. Not knowing how things will turn out can trigger anxiety. To navigate uncertainty:

1. **Practice Mindfulness**: Stay in the present moment rather than speculating about worst-case scenarios. Simple breathing or meditation techniques can ground you.
2. **Develop Contingency Plans**: If you have a Plan A, consider a Plan B. This does not mean you are pessimistic; it means you are prepared.
3. **Focus on Values**: When external circumstances are shaky, your core values remain stable. Let those values guide your decisions. For instance, if you value family, you will prioritize them even if your job situation changes.

Recognizing that uncertainty is normal can also provide comfort. No one can predict every outcome, so compassion for yourself is vital.

## Finding Meaning in Change

Some life challenges—like a serious illness or losing a loved one—can be devastating, and it is natural to feel grief or anger. While you cannot always see a bright side in such events, over time, you may find meaning in the way you respond to them.

- **Reprioritizing**: A health scare might lead you to focus more on fitness or enjoying time with family.

- **Empathy for Others**: If you have endured a tough experience, you might become more empathetic or supportive to friends going through similar trials.
- **Personal Transformation**: Some individuals emerge from hardships with a clearer sense of purpose or newfound strengths they never knew they had.

This does not justify or diminish the pain you have gone through. Rather, it acknowledges that the human spirit is capable of growth even in darkness.

---

## Embracing Reinvention

At times, change calls for a major reinvention of who you are. Maybe you shift from a corporate career to becoming a teacher, or you go from being single to parenting multiple children. Embrace the fact that your identity can expand. You can carry forward lessons from your old life into the new one, blending past experiences with future possibilities.

**Tips for Reinvention**:

- **Compile Transferable Skills**: Think about skills you have developed in one role that could apply to another. For instance, leadership in an office could translate to heading community initiatives.
- **Clarify Your New Vision**: Journaling or vision boards can help you see how you want your life to look after the change.
- **Be Willing to Let Go**: Holding onto old ways of thinking or old goals might stunt your growth. Recognize which aspects of your past no longer serve who you are becoming.

Reinvention is not about erasing your old self; it is about evolving to meet new circumstances with creativity and resilience.

---

## Handling Relapses into Old Patterns

Even after you have adapted, stressful moments or reminders can pull you back into old habits. Maybe you handle a career shift well but feel waves of anxiety if you see a job listing similar to your old position. This is normal. Adaptation is not a linear process—it can zigzag.

- **Self-Awareness**: Stay alert to triggers that cause you to doubt or revert to outdated thinking.
- **Revisit Coping Techniques**: Reapply the strategies that helped you adapt in the first place, like journaling, talking with a mentor, or restructuring your daily routine.
- **Acknowledge Progress**: You are not the same person you were before the change. List the ways you have grown to remind yourself of how far you have come.

Slip-ups in mindset do not invalidate your overall transformation. They are just signals that you may need to reaffirm your new approach.

---

## Celebrating Milestones in Adaptation

One overlooked part of adapting is pausing to recognize your achievements. Did you finally settle into a new job and feel confident after months of training? Celebrate that. Did you finish moving into your new home and build a sense of comfort? Acknowledge it. Celebrations do not have to be extravagant. Even a small treat or a heartfelt journal entry can mark the moment you realize you have come through a challenge stronger and wiser.

# Chapter 17: Leadership and Influence

## Introduction

You do not need a fancy title or a huge following to be a leader. True leadership is about inspiring, guiding, and empowering others. You can lead in your family, your workplace, your community, or online. In this chapter, we will focus on what leadership really means, how you can learn to influence people in positive ways, and why women often bring unique strengths to leadership roles. By the end, you will see that leadership is not about trying to be the "boss" of everyone. It is about using your talents and values to make a difference in the world around you.

## What Is Leadership?

Leadership is the ability to motivate people toward a shared goal. It involves setting a direction and encouraging others to follow. But it also means listening to those you lead, learning from them, and adapting as needed. Effective leaders do not simply issue orders; they also show empathy, open-mindedness, and consistency.

### Qualities of Good Leaders

- **Integrity**: Being honest and standing by your principles, even when no one is watching.
- **Empathy**: Understanding people's feelings, challenges, and perspectives.
- **Vision**: Having a clear idea of what you want to achieve.
- **Communication**: Sharing your ideas effectively and listening attentively.
- **Adaptability**: Being flexible when faced with changes or obstacles.
- **Courage**: Willingness to take risks and make tough decisions.

Not every leader starts out with all these qualities. Many of them develop over time through practice, mistakes, and learning from challenges.

## Formal vs. Informal Leadership

Some leadership roles are formal, like when you are elected as a committee chair at work or become the head of an organization. You have a recognized title and specific responsibilities. But informal leadership is just as important. You may be the one people turn to for advice, the one who organizes group outings, or the person who quietly inspires others with your actions. Both types can create meaningful impact.

## Leading with Your Own Style

There is no single "correct" way to lead. Some people are naturally outgoing and like to speak up in big groups. Others lead through one-on-one mentoring or quietly setting examples. You might be someone who enjoys strategic planning and data analysis, or you might excel at building personal connections. The key is to embrace your strengths and be authentic. When you try to mimic someone else's style, you risk seeming insincere and losing your unique spark.

## Building Trust and Credibility

People follow those they trust. Without trust, even the best ideas can fail to gain support. Trust is earned by keeping your promises, being consistent, and showing respect. When you make a mistake, acknowledge it rather than hiding it. This honesty shows you are human and willing to learn, which often makes people trust you more, not less.

**Simple Ways to Build Trust**

1. **Do What You Say**: If you promise to complete a task by Friday, do so—or communicate early if you need extra time.
2. **Show Respect**: Listen fully when someone shares an idea, even if you disagree.
3. **Admit Mistakes**: Own up to errors and focus on making them right.
4. **Keep Private Matters Private**: If someone shares sensitive information, do not gossip about it.

Trust can be destroyed quickly if you break your word or misuse someone's confidence. Protect it like a valuable asset.

## Communication: Listening and Speaking Clearly

Effective communication is the backbone of leadership. You need to share your goals or vision so others understand where you are heading. But you also need to listen—often more than you speak. Good leaders ask questions, pay attention to the answers, and adapt their approach when they realize there is a misunderstanding.

- **Clarity**: Use simple language when explaining what you want to do or why you want to do it. Avoid vague phrases that confuse people.
- **Active Listening**: Give your full focus to the person speaking. Do not just wait for your turn to talk.
- **Constructive Feedback**: When you need to correct someone, be gentle yet direct. Focus on the behavior, not their worth as a person.

## Empathy and Understanding Others

Being empathetic does not mean you ignore problems or accept poor performance. It means you try to understand why someone might be struggling or upset. Maybe a coworker is distracted because of a family issue. Maybe a team member is shy and hates speaking in large groups. By noticing these things, you can offer support or adapt tasks in ways that help them succeed. Empathy builds loyalty and helps you bring out the best in others.

## Leading Through Challenges

Leadership shines most during difficult times. When problems arise, people look to leaders for guidance, reassurance, and solutions. You do not need all the answers at once. What matters is staying calm, thinking clearly, and showing you are willing to take steps forward.

- **Keep Communication Open**: Let people know what is happening, even if you do not have a final solution yet.
- **Delegate and Collaborate**: You do not have to fix everything yourself. Ask others for ideas.
- **Stay Flexible**: If one approach fails, pivot to another. Being stubborn rarely helps solve big problems.

Leading through hardship can test your resilience. It can also build your credibility if you remain honest, composed, and solution-focused.

## Influence vs. Manipulation

Influence is about persuading or inspiring others in a positive, honest way. Manipulation involves tricking or pressuring people to do what you want, often by withholding facts or playing on their fears. While manipulation can bring short-term results, it damages trust and morale in the long run. Leaders who rely on manipulation often lose respect over time.

### Positive Influence

- **Model Good Behavior**: Be the example you want others to follow.
- **Explain the "Why"**: People are more engaged when they know why a task matters.
- **Share Credit**: If something goes well, acknowledge the team's contributions. This encourages people to keep supporting you.

## Women and Leadership

For a long time, women were not given the same leadership opportunities as men in many cultures. Thankfully, this is changing, but certain barriers and biases still exist. Women in leadership may face extra scrutiny or be labeled as "too bossy" when they act assertively. Understanding these societal pressures can help you find ways to lead confidently without shrinking yourself to fit outdated expectations.

- **Speak Up for Yourself**: Clearly express your ideas, set boundaries, and do not apologize for having authority or knowledge.
- **Seek Allies**: Find mentors, sponsors, or peers who understand your challenges and will support your growth.
- **Stay True to Your Style**: You do not have to adopt stereotypically "male" behavior to be an effective leader. Use the unique strengths you bring—such as empathy, collaboration, or creativity.

## Everyday Leadership Opportunities

You do not need a big title to practice leadership. Look for smaller openings in daily life:

- **Family**: Organize a family meeting to plan activities or address conflicts. Guide discussions to ensure everyone feels heard.
- **Work or School**: Volunteer to lead a project or host a brainstorming session.
- **Community**: Offer your skills at local events, like a charity drive or a neighborhood clean-up. Take charge of certain tasks or suggest improvements.
- **Online Spaces**: If you run a social media group or blog, set a positive tone, moderate discussions fairly, and encourage open dialogue.

In each of these settings, use what you have learned about empathy, communication, and ethics. Over time, your influence grows.

## Dealing with Criticism and Conflict

Leadership inevitably means facing criticism or conflict. Someone might dislike your plan, feel overshadowed, or simply have a different opinion. Your response to this criticism can either escalate tensions or move toward resolution.

- **Stay Calm**: If you respond with anger, the conflict usually intensifies.
- **Listen Actively**: Hear the person out. Sometimes there is a useful point in their criticism.
- **Seek Solutions**: Work together to find a middle ground. If compromise is not possible, explain your reasoning respectfully.
- **Maintain Respect**: Even if you disagree strongly, do not resort to personal attacks.

Criticism can be an opportunity to learn, refine your approach, or affirm that you are on the right path (if the criticism is unfounded). A good leader shows they can handle opposing views with grace.

## Public Speaking and Presentation

Being able to speak clearly in front of others is a valuable leadership skill. This does not mean you have to love public speaking, but practicing basic techniques can boost your influence:

- **Know Your Points**: Outline your main ideas. People remember clear, structured messages.

- **Practice**: Run through your talk a few times, noting where you stumble or lose the thread.
- **Engage the Audience**: Make eye contact, ask questions, or invite brief feedback. People listen more if they feel involved.
- **Be Authentic**: If you are naturally serious, do not force humor. If you are lively, do not hide that energy. Being genuine helps you connect with people.

Even if you are nervous, learning how to speak confidently can help you advocate for your ideas and inspire others to join you.

## Leading Yourself First

Before effectively leading others, you need to lead yourself. This means having self-discipline, emotional intelligence, and personal accountability. If you cannot manage your own time, stress, or behaviors, it becomes harder to guide others. Leading yourself includes:

- **Setting Personal Goals**: Know what you want to achieve in your own life.
- **Practicing Self-Care**: Keep your mind and body healthy, as discussed in previous chapters.
- **Reflecting on Actions**: Think about what went well and what you could improve in your daily interactions.
- **Staying Open to Feedback**: If you are wrong, admit it and work to do better.

When you show that you can manage yourself responsibly, people trust you to manage tasks, projects, and even communities.

## Long-Term Leadership Development

Leadership is not a one-time skill but an ongoing journey. Even experienced leaders keep learning. To grow over the long term:

1. **Stay Curious**: Read books on leadership, communication, and problem-solving. Watch talks by influential leaders.
2. **Attend Workshops or Classes**: Many organizations offer leadership training programs.

3. **Seek Mentors**: Find someone with experience and watch how they handle different situations. Ask for feedback on your own approach.
4. **Reflect Regularly**: Keep a journal to track your leadership experiences—the wins, the challenges, and the lessons.

Embrace the idea that leadership styles can change as you do. You might be more hands-on at the start of your career, then become more of a mentor later. Adapt your style to fit your growth and the needs of those you lead.

# Chapter 18: Financial Independence and Responsibility

## Introduction

Money is not everything, but it does shape many aspects of our lives. Whether you want to pursue education, start a family, travel, or build a business, having a stable financial foundation can make these goals more accessible. Financial independence means you have enough resources to live without constant worry, and financial responsibility means you manage money wisely to maintain or improve your situation.

In this chapter, we will explore the basics of budgeting, saving, debt management, and investing—key skills for any woman looking to take charge of her financial future. By understanding these concepts, you can reduce stress about money and free up mental space to focus on other areas of personal growth.

## Why Financial Independence Matters

Financial independence is not just about being rich; it is about having the freedom to make life choices based on personal values rather than financial constraints. For some, it might mean being able to leave a toxic job or an unhealthy relationship. For others, it could be saving for a child's education or starting a small business. Financial independence gives you options and reduces feelings of powerlessness.

## Budgeting: The Foundation of Financial Health

A budget is a simple plan for how you will use the money that comes in and goes out. It helps you see where you might be wasting funds and where you could reallocate them toward your goals. Budgeting can feel tedious at first, but it becomes second nature once you see the benefits.

**Steps to Create a Basic Budget**

1. **Track Your Income**: Note all your income sources—salary, side gigs, rental income, etc.
2. **List Expenses**: Write down monthly costs such as rent, utilities, groceries, and any debts.
3. **Set Saving Goals**: Decide how much you want to save or invest every month. Treat this like a non-negotiable bill to yourself.
4. **Identify "Leakage"**: Look for areas where money is unnecessarily spent (e.g., subscriptions you do not use).
5. **Adjust and Monitor**: Fine-tune your budget each month. You might discover you need to reduce certain expenses or that you can afford to save more.

Many people find budgeting apps or spreadsheets helpful, but even a plain notebook can work. The key is consistency—check your budget regularly to ensure you are on track.

## Building an Emergency Fund

An emergency fund is a savings account set aside for unexpected costs—like car repairs, medical bills, or urgent home maintenance. Aim to save three to six months' worth of living expenses, if possible. Start small if needed, but make it a priority. Having this cushion gives you peace of mind and prevents a sudden crisis from plunging you into debt.

## Understanding and Managing Debt

Debt itself is not always bad. A mortgage on a house or a student loan to improve your skills can be worthwhile investments. However, high-interest consumer debt—like credit card balances that are not paid in full—can become a financial burden.

- **Pay More Than the Minimum**: If you only pay the minimum on credit cards, you might be stuck in a cycle for years.
- **Prioritize High-Interest Debt**: Focus on paying off debts with the highest interest rate first, as that saves you the most money over time.
- **Consider Debt Consolidation**: Combining multiple debts into one loan with a lower interest rate can make repayment more manageable.

If your debt feels overwhelming, speak with a financial counselor or a reputable nonprofit organization. Avoid quick-fix schemes that promise to erase debt without proper explanation; they often lead to worse problems.

## Saving and Investing

Saving is putting aside money to use in the future, while investing involves using that money to potentially grow your wealth. Both are important steps on the road to financial independence.

### Different Savings Buckets

- **Emergency Fund**: Already discussed—your first priority.
- **Short-Term Goals**: Maybe you want a vacation or a new computer. Keep this money somewhere easily accessible, such as a savings account.
- **Long-Term Goals**: Retirement, buying a home, or funding a business. These might require more strategic investment choices.

### Investing Basics

Investing means putting your money into assets—like stocks, bonds, mutual funds, or real estate—that could grow in value over time. It comes with risks, but historically, investing has yielded higher returns than simply letting money sit in a regular bank account. If you are new to investing, start by learning the basics:

1. **Risk and Return**: Higher potential returns usually come with higher risk.
2. **Diversification**: "Do not put all your eggs in one basket." Spread your money across different types of investments.
3. **Time Horizon**: The longer you keep your investments, the more you can ride out market ups and downs.
4. **Retirement Accounts**: In many countries, there are special retirement accounts (like 401(k) or IRA in the U.S.) that offer tax advantages. Look into what is available in your region.

It helps to read up on finance basics, watch tutorials, or consult a certified financial planner if possible. Even small monthly contributions to an investment account can grow significantly over time due to compound interest.

## Financial Goals and Milestones

Setting clear goals keeps you motivated. Maybe you want to pay off a student loan within five years or save enough for a down payment on a home. Break these goals into milestones, such as paying off 20% of the debt by a certain date or saving a certain percentage of your monthly income.

Each time you reach a milestone—like clearing a debt or accumulating a particular amount in savings—celebrate in a modest way. Small rewards reinforce positive habits, but be sure they do not undo your progress (avoid throwing a big party that puts you back into debt).

## Negotiating and Asking for What You Are Worth

Women historically have been paid less than men in many regions, partly because they are less likely to negotiate salaries or raises. Learning to negotiate is a valuable skill that can improve your financial security.

- **Research Market Rates**: Know the average salary for your position and level of experience.
- **List Achievements**: Gather evidence of your contributions—projects led, money saved for the company, positive feedback from clients.
- **Practice**: Role-play with a friend or mentor to get comfortable stating your desired salary or rate.
- **Stay Confident and Polite**: Negotiation does not have to be confrontational. Calmly present your data and be open to discussion.

If your request is denied, ask for clear feedback or other forms of compensation, such as flexible hours, extra vacation days, or professional development funding.

## Protecting Your Financial Future

Aside from saving and investing, consider other protective measures:

- **Insurance**: Health, life, disability, and property insurance can shield you from huge financial losses if something goes wrong.
- **Estate Planning**: If you have assets or dependents, it is wise to have a simple will or trust, and instructions for healthcare decisions if you become unable to speak for yourself.

- **Identity Theft Prevention**: Monitor bank statements, use strong passwords, and be cautious when sharing personal information online.

While these measures seem tedious, they create a safety net that guards the progress you have worked hard to build.

## Everyday Money Habits

Financial responsibility is not only about big decisions like mortgages or investments. Daily habits also play a significant role. Examples:

- **Live Within Your Means**: Try not to spend more than you earn. This principle, though simple, is often overlooked.
- **Avoid Impulse Purchases**: Take a moment to think, "Do I really need this?" before buying something non-essential.
- **Use Cash or Debit When Possible**: Paying with physical money can make you more aware of spending than swiping a card.
- **Plan Meals and Shop Smart**: Cooking at home, using a grocery list, and buying in bulk for items you use often can save a lot over time.

These everyday practices align with your bigger goals of saving, paying off debt, or investing.

## Overcoming Emotional Spending

It is common to use shopping or spending as a way to cope with stress, sadness, or even boredom. While a small treat now and then can be fine, repeated emotional spending can derail your budget.

- **Identify Triggers**: Notice when you tend to shop impulsively—after a bad day at work or a conflict with a friend.
- **Find Alternatives**: Instead of shopping online to lift your mood, try going for a walk, writing in a journal, or calling a supportive friend.
- **Set Boundaries**: Give yourself a 24-hour rule before making non-essential purchases. This pause often reduces impulse buys.

By managing emotional spending, you gain better control over where your money goes and keep your finances aligned with your real needs and goals.

## Supporting Others Without Sacrificing Yourself

Women often feel pressured to help friends or family financially, sometimes beyond their means. While generosity is admirable, be mindful of your own security. If you are asked for money or to co-sign loans, think carefully:

- **Check Your Budget**: Can you truly afford to give this amount without harming your goals?
- **Discuss Expectations**: Is the money a gift or a loan? If it is a loan, how will it be repaid?
- **Balance Empathy and Reality**: You want to help, but if giving money puts your own stability at risk, you could end up needing help yourself.

It is okay to say "no" or offer smaller support if you cannot afford a larger request. Healthy boundaries protect your financial future.

## Financial Independence as a Path to Empowerment

Having control over your finances can boost self-esteem and reduce anxiety. It lets you make choices based on your dreams rather than on sheer necessity. Financially independent women can leave bad relationships, survive job loss, or fund children's education without feeling trapped by lack of resources.

Additionally, economic power often translates into a louder voice in community and policy matters. When women have money, they can invest in local businesses, sponsor scholarships, or donate to causes they believe in, further amplifying their influence and leadership.

## Long-Term Vision

Financial independence is not usually achieved overnight. It requires patience and consistent effort. Whether you are working on paying off high-interest debt, building an investment portfolio, or saving for a special project, keep your eyes on the bigger picture. Revisit your goals regularly, celebrate small successes, and adjust when life circumstances change.

# Chapter 19: Building Emotional Resilience

## Introduction

Life is full of emotional ups and downs. At times, you may feel overjoyed and positive, while other times, stress, heartbreak, or unexpected problems can leave you feeling overwhelmed. **Emotional resilience** is the ability to bounce back from these hardships and continue moving forward—learning from the pain rather than letting it crush your spirit.

You have already explored topics like self-care, managing stress, and overcoming fears in earlier chapters. Here, we will focus on how to deepen your emotional resilience in new ways. This means developing the mental and emotional "muscles" that help you cope with challenges and emerge stronger. By the end, you will see that resilience does not mean never feeling upset or hurt; rather, it is about not staying down forever when life knocks you off your feet.

---

## What Is Emotional Resilience?

Emotional resilience is the capacity to handle life's emotional blows without losing your sense of self or hope. It does not mean you never cry or feel afraid. Instead, it means you eventually recover and learn something useful from each struggle. Think of it like a rubber band that can stretch under pressure but not break—returning to its original shape once the tension eases.

### Signs of Emotional Resilience

- You can experience sadness or stress but eventually regain calm or optimism.
- You are comfortable seeking help or talking about your feelings rather than bottling them up.
- You learn lessons from tough experiences instead of merely suffering through them.

- You believe you can handle future challenges because you have handled difficulties before.

Anyone can become more resilient with practice, no matter how fragile you might feel today. It is not an all-or-nothing trait; it grows through each test life throws at you.

---

## Common Blocks to Resilience

Sometimes, we unintentionally hold onto habits or beliefs that weaken our resilience. These can include:

- **Long-Term Self-Doubt**: Constantly telling yourself you cannot handle problems makes it harder to move past them.
- **Fear of Vulnerability**: Believing that showing emotion or asking for help is a sign of weakness can keep you from receiving the support you need.
- **Ruminating on Past Hurts**: Continuously replaying old pain in your head can trap you in negative emotions instead of letting you look ahead.

Recognizing these blocks is the first step toward building better coping strategies. Once you see how these mindsets drag you down, you can start untying them so you can become more flexible and strong emotionally.

---

## The Role of Self-Awareness

A big part of emotional resilience is recognizing your own emotional patterns. Instead of labeling your feelings as purely good or bad, try to see them as signals. If you feel anxious every time you get a new work assignment, for instance, that may point to underlying self-doubt or fear of failure. Instead of ignoring these signals, use them as clues about where you can grow.

**Small Self-Awareness Practices**

- **Emotional Check-Ins**: Pause once or twice a day to name what you are feeling—happy, tense, frustrated, hopeful. Understanding how you feel is the first step to managing it.

- **Ask "Why?"**: When a strong emotion arises, gently ask yourself why. For example, if you are suddenly irritable, you might discover you are overwhelmed by a tight schedule. This allows you to adjust and regain control.
- **Journaling**: Even a few short sentences each day can help you notice emotional trends, such as repeated frustration in certain situations.

Gaining self-awareness does not stop negative emotions from ever popping up. Instead, it helps you address them more quickly and choose helpful responses rather than knee-jerk reactions.

## Healthy Release of Emotions

Resilience does not mean bottling up your sadness, anger, or fear. In fact, repressed emotions can grow stronger over time and burst out in harmful ways. Instead, find healthy methods to release emotions so they do not linger and poison your outlook:

- **Gentle Expression**: Cry if you need to, talk it out with a trusted friend, or write down your feelings privately.
- **Physical Outlets**: Light exercise, a brisk walk, or dancing to music you enjoy can help burn off the physical tension associated with stress or anger.
- **Creative Channels**: Draw, paint, sing, or craft something that captures your mood. This transforms difficult feelings into a creative process rather than letting them stay stuck.

Giving yourself permission to feel and release emotions in a safe way prevents them from piling up like a hidden weight on your shoulders.

## Challenging Harmful Thought Patterns

Negative self-talk often weakens resilience. If a stressful event occurs and you respond by thinking, "I can't deal with this," or "I'm a total failure," you may spiral into despair. Instead, practice reframing these thoughts.

- **Original Thought**: "I always ruin everything."
- **Reframe**: "I made a mistake this time, but I can fix it or handle the fallout."

This mental shift does not erase the problem, but it keeps your sense of self-worth intact and maintains hope that solutions exist. You are training your mind to be flexible rather than rigid under stress, which supports resilience.

---

## Finding Meaning in Challenges

Sometimes, the hardships we face can lead us to question why they happened. Searching for meaning does not necessarily mean finding a grand reason for suffering, but it does encourage you to see what lessons or strengths might come from the experience.

- **Deepened Empathy**: Going through heartbreak can make you more compassionate toward others facing similar pain.
- **Clarified Priorities**: A major illness can highlight which relationships or dreams truly matter to you.
- **New Directions**: Losing a job might push you to explore a career path that aligns better with your passions and values.

While no one wants to experience heartbreak or loss, seeing potential silver linings can help you cope and eventually emerge stronger.

---

## Strengthening Your Support System

Resilience does not develop in isolation. Having a network of trustworthy people—friends, family members, mentors, or support groups—offers a cushion when life delivers a blow. Even a simple conversation with someone who cares can remind you that you are not alone in your struggles.

- **Choose Support Wisely**: Share sensitive struggles with those who have proven trustworthy, not just anyone.
- **Offer and Accept Help**: A resilient mindset includes the humility to accept help and the generosity to give it when you can. Both acts deepen human bonds.

- **Stay Connected**: Make time for meaningful interactions, whether a phone call, a quick coffee, or a supportive text message.

Knowing you have supportive people standing by can lessen the fear that you must tackle every hardship alone.

---

## Building Optimism and Hope

Emotional resilience is closely tied to an optimistic outlook. Again, this is not about denying reality or ignoring problems; it is about trusting that you can find ways to move forward.

- **Remind Yourself of Past Victories**: Recall times when you overcame difficulties or learned valuable lessons from failure. This reflection builds confidence.
- **Celebrate Small Joys**: Even during a crisis, brief moments of happiness—like enjoying a beautiful sunset or hearing a friend's laughter—can remind you that life still holds positive experiences.
- **Look Ahead**: Rather than dwelling on what went wrong, try to imagine a future where you have found solutions or adapted to new circumstances.

In tough periods, optimism can feel forced, but practicing it consistently teaches your mind to see possibilities instead of dead ends.

---

## Emotional Boundaries in Relationships

Part of resilience involves protecting your emotional energy. If certain relationships constantly drag you into drama or sadness, they may hinder your ability to stay strong. Setting boundaries does not mean cutting people off at the first sign of trouble; it means recognizing how much emotional energy you can give without harming yourself.

- **Know Your Limits**: If you find yourself drained after certain interactions, consider limiting the time or changing the conversation topics.
- **Communicate Calmly**: Explain your boundaries if needed, such as saying, "I'm not comfortable discussing this topic today, but I appreciate your understanding."

- **Seek Balance**: Healthy relationships should involve give-and-take, not just one person pouring out emotional support without receiving any.

Maintaining emotional boundaries keeps you from being overwhelmed, allowing you to remain resilient.

---

## Facing Fear and Anxiety with Courage

Fear can paralyze resilience if you let it. Whether you are afraid of failing, looking foolish, or facing an unknown future, the key is to take small steps to confront what scares you.

- **Gradual Exposure**: If public speaking terrifies you, start by practicing with a friend, then a small group, before presenting at a large event.
- **Stay in the Present**: Anxiety often focuses on what might happen. Ground yourself in current reality—what is happening right now, and what can you do in this moment?
- **Acknowledge Accomplishments**: Each time you face a fear, you prove to yourself that you can do hard things. Celebrate these moments, no matter how small.

Meeting your fears head-on teaches you that they do not have absolute power over you, which strengthens emotional resilience for future challenges.

---

## Mindful Approaches to Stress

You have learned various stress-management tools in previous chapters, but let us consider adding a mindful twist. Instead of just trying to calm down, **mindful stress management** involves truly noticing and naming your stress. Example: "I feel my stomach twisting, my breathing is shallow, and my mind is racing." By describing the sensations without judgment, you may notice they lose some of their intensity.

- **Moment of Pause**: If something triggers high stress, pause for a few deep breaths and observe your physical state.

- **Soothing Words**: Gently tell yourself, "I see you are stressed. You can handle this one step at a time."
- **Return to Action**: After acknowledging the stress, take the next small action, such as writing down your top priority or making a phone call for help.

This mindful approach prevents stress from piling up unnoticed and helps you respond thoughtfully rather than impulsively.

---

## Resilience and Self-Compassion

Being tough on yourself when you fail does not build resilience—it often shatters it. Self-compassion is the understanding that you deserve kindness, especially when you are struggling or have made mistakes.

- **Imagine a Kind Friend**: If you are tempted to scold yourself, think about how you would comfort a dear friend in the same situation. Use those words on yourself.
- **Gentle Self-Talk**: Instead of "I'm so stupid for letting this happen," try "I'm disappointed this happened, but I can learn and move forward."
- **Accept Imperfection**: Even resilient people slip up. Recognize that being flawed is part of being human.

Self-compassion gives you a stable emotional base from which you can rebuild and grow.

---

## Putting Resilience into Daily Practice

Building emotional resilience is an ongoing process, not a one-time event. Consider adding small rituals to your everyday routine:

1. **Morning Check-In**: Spend a minute each morning asking yourself how you feel. If you sense tension or worry, plan a calming activity for later, like a short walk or a moment of quiet reflection.

2. **Midday Encouragement**: During a lunch break or a quick pause, remind yourself of one thing you are handling well. A little boost can keep your momentum up through the afternoon.
3. **Evening Reflection**: Before bed, think of one challenge you faced that day. Did you handle it in a resilient manner? If so, applaud yourself. If not, note one small change you could try next time.

These simple acts keep the concept of resilience fresh in your mind and help you track your emotional growth over time.

## Recognizing Your Progress

Emotional resilience is often easiest to see in hindsight. Maybe you realize that last year, you would have panicked over a minor work crisis, but today you dealt with it calmly. Or perhaps you used to hold grudges for months, but now you address conflicts and move on more quickly.

- **Celebrate Victories**: Each time you handle a tough situation without falling apart is a win worth acknowledging.
- **Track Patterns**: Notice if your recovery time after disappointments is shorter. That is a sign of growing resilience.
- **Offer Gratitude**: Thank yourself for putting in the effort to grow. Gratitude can be directed inward, too.

Recognizing progress reinforces your belief that resilience can be cultivated. The next time life challenges you, you can recall these improvements and trust that you have the emotional skills to persevere.

# Chapter 20: Sustaining Growth and Next Steps

## Introduction

Over the course of this book, you have gone through a journey—from discovering your true self to building confidence, juggling family and personal space, nurturing relationships, taking care of your mind and body, expanding your creativity, shaping a positive mindset, adapting to change, and more. You have learned that personal growth is multi-layered and ongoing.

In this final chapter, we will bring everything together. You will explore how to maintain the progress you have made, keep challenging yourself, and remain open to life's new phases and twists. Sustaining growth means recognizing that self-improvement is not a one-time event; it is a lifelong process, and each step builds on the last.

---

### Reflecting on How Far You Have Come

Before rushing ahead, pause to see what you have already achieved. It is easy to get stuck chasing the next goal without celebrating small or large successes. Reflecting on your progress provides motivation to continue.

- **Look Back at Old Struggles**: Are you handling any of those better now? Maybe fear does not hold you back as much, or you speak up for yourself more often.
- **Review Your Journals or Notes**: If you have been writing about your journey, compare older entries with recent ones. Notice shifts in your mindset or accomplishments you forgot you had.
- **Acknowledge Growth in Relationships**: Perhaps certain relationships are less tense, or you have established firmer but healthier boundaries.

Seeing these improvements helps you realize that all the effort was worthwhile—and that you can keep going.

## Setting New Goals and Adventures

Personal growth does not end; it evolves. After you have tackled your initial goals—like gaining confidence or managing your finances—it might be time to branch out or aim higher. Setting new goals can keep life exciting and push you beyond the comfort zone you have established.

- **Skill Expansion**: If you mastered basic financial management, maybe you now explore investing or entrepreneurship. If you became healthier physically, you could try a new sport or a hiking challenge.
- **Creative Projects**: If you discovered a passion for art or writing, consider a bigger project, like a short story collection or a community art show.
- **Community Involvement**: Maybe you decide to volunteer for a local cause, serve on a board, or mentor young people in your field.

Choose goals that align with your personal values, so your motivation comes naturally. Goals that excite you on a deeper level are more likely to stick than those you pursue just because you "should."

---

## Maintaining Balance

As you continue to grow, it is crucial to maintain balance in your life. Hyper-focusing on one aspect—like work success—can strain relationships or health if you are not careful. Recall the lessons about setting boundaries and watching for signs of burnout. A fulfilling life is not about perfect equilibrium at every moment, but about noticing when one area is taking too much and adjusting accordingly.

- **Regular Check-Ins**: Schedule moments (monthly or quarterly) to ask yourself if any part of your life feels neglected—health, family, personal passions, spiritual practices, or something else.
- **Adapt Boundaries**: As your responsibilities shift—maybe you get a promotion or have a second child—your time and energy availability will change. Adjust boundaries or routines as needed.
- **Prioritize Rest and Leisure**: Growth includes knowing when to pause. Resting your mind and body keeps you from depleting yourself, allowing room for new ideas and continued enthusiasm.

Staying balanced ensures you do not lose sight of all-around well-being while chasing the next goal.

## Embracing Lifelong Learning

One of the most powerful tools for ongoing growth is a mindset of continuous learning. This does not necessarily mean formal education; it can be as simple as reading a book on a topic you know little about, watching documentaries, or practicing a new hobby. Learning keeps your brain active and flexible, traits that support growth in every area of life.

- **Stay Curious**: Ask questions about things you see or hear. Look up new terms, explore different cultures, or challenge yourself to try something unfamiliar.
- **Find Inspiring Mentors**: Seek out individuals you admire—either in your personal network or through interviews, articles, or online platforms. Learn from their experiences and insights.
- **Share Knowledge**: Teaching what you know is also a form of learning. When you explain a concept to someone else, you reinforce your own understanding and possibly spark new ideas.

Lifelong learning ensures you remain adaptable and open-minded, ready to handle whatever changes come your way.

## Monitoring and Adjusting Your Mindset

You have discovered the importance of a positive, growth-oriented mindset. Yet even the most optimistic people can backslide into doubts or negativity under stress. Periodically assess where your thoughts are trending. Are you allowing negative self-talk to creep back in? Are you returning to a fixed mindset when you face a new challenge?

- **Affirmations and Visual Reminders**: Place uplifting quotes or personal mantras where you can see them daily. These small nudges can keep your mind from slipping into a negative loop.

- **Self-Talk Audits**: Catch yourself if you start saying things like "I can't do this" or "I'm not good enough." Pause and rephrase your thoughts: "This is tough, but I can learn" or "I'll try a different strategy."
- **Celebrate Progress**: Even if you are not at your final goal, noticing incremental improvements helps you stay motivated and counters pessimism.

Mindset maintenance is an ongoing process, but each tune-up keeps you from drifting too far off course.

---

## Continuing to Nurture Relationships

Healthy relationships with friends, family, and romantic partners require regular care. As you grow personally, your relationships may shift. Some individuals might be thrilled by your progress; others might feel threatened or left behind. By openly communicating and inviting loved ones to learn and grow with you, you can keep your bonds strong or form new, uplifting connections.

- **Share Your Journey**: Tell people you trust about your new goals or achievements, so they understand the changes in your life. This can deepen closeness and respect.
- **Stay Open to Feedback**: Loved ones might see areas of improvement you have missed. Be open-minded if they gently suggest ways you could handle situations better.
- **Give Support Back**: As you gain more confidence and knowledge, offer it to those around you who might be struggling. Being supportive reinforces your own growth principles.

Maintaining strong, supportive relationships acts as a buffer against future stressors and helps you continue evolving.

---

## Periodic Self-Evaluation

One way to ensure you keep growing is to schedule self-evaluations. This is not about criticizing yourself harshly; it is about checking in with honesty and compassion. Once or twice a year, sit down with a notebook and think about:

1. **Wins and Milestones**: What did you accomplish since your last evaluation? Big or small, list them all to remind yourself of your progress.
2. **Areas of Struggle**: Where did you stumble or backtrack? What kept you from moving forward in certain domains—health, finances, creativity, relationships, or mental well-being?
3. **Lessons Learned**: Each struggle or success likely taught you something. Write down these lessons explicitly.
4. **Next Goals**: Based on what you have learned, what do you want to focus on for the next six to twelve months?

These reflective sessions help you remain mindful and intentional about your life's direction. You can spot patterns—like always procrastinating on financial tasks or neglecting your self-care routine when work gets hectic—and plan solutions.

---

## Embracing Change and Uncertainty

Earlier chapters addressed handling change and building resilience. As you keep growing, do not assume life will become smooth forever. New chapters, new goals, and new external events will challenge you again. Rather than fear the unknown, accept it as a chance to test your new skills and discover further strengths.

- **Stay Flexible**: Plans might shift due to factors outside your control, like economic shifts or health issues. Adjust where you can, maintaining your core values and determination.
- **Apply Resilience Tools**: When unexpected stress hits, remember you have already gained coping strategies—breathing techniques, journaling, boundary-setting, or reaching out to trusted supporters.
- **Trust Your Growth**: Even if you do not see immediate solutions, you can believe in your ability to figure things out, step by step.

Every challenge is an opportunity to reaffirm that you are not the same person you were before—you have grown and can continue to do so.

## Sharing Your Growth with the World

At some point, you may feel a desire to give back or share what you have learned. This could be as simple as mentoring a younger colleague, volunteering, or starting a small group in your community focused on personal development topics. When you share your experiences, you help others find their path while also solidifying your own lessons.

- **Mentoring**: Offer guidance to someone who is a few steps behind you. Listening to their struggles can remind you of your own journey and how you overcame similar hurdles.
- **Public Speaking or Workshops**: If you feel comfortable, host small workshops—online or in-person—on topics like building confidence, managing stress, or setting healthy boundaries.
- **Content Creation**: Some people create blogs, podcasts, or social media groups. This can spread encouragement to a wider audience, although it is optional.

Contributing to others' growth multiplies the impact of your own efforts, creating a ripple effect of positivity and empowerment.

---

## Letting Go of Perfection

Even with solid plans and a strong sense of self, you will never be perfectly "done" with growth. Perfectionism can creep in, causing stress and guilt if you do not meet every expectation. Remind yourself:

- **Growth is a Process**: You are constantly in motion, learning from each new experience.
- **Mistakes Are Part of the Journey**: Nobody grows without stumbling at times. Each mistake offers lessons.
- **Self-Compassion is Key**: When you do not achieve a goal on time, allow yourself to be human. Reassess, adjust, and move on.

Accepting imperfection frees you to keep trying without the fear of failing. It also helps you enjoy the journey rather than always pushing toward a never-ending finish line.

## Making Peace with Rest and Slow Periods

There will be seasons in life when everything feels dynamic—new ideas, new achievements, rapid progress. But other times, you might feel stuck or just less driven. Understand that not every moment of life is meant for huge breakthroughs. Some phases are for resting, healing, or quietly processing what you have learned.

- **Value Slower Times**: This is when your mind can integrate lessons, and your body can recharge.
- **Tune In to Your Energy**: If you sense you are burned out, take a short hiatus from big goals. Focus on smaller tasks or restful activities.
- **Trust the Cycle**: After a dormant period, you may naturally feel ready to push forward again. This cycle mirrors nature's seasons—growth, bloom, harvest, rest.

Accepting these ebbs and flows prevents burnout and makes each active phase more productive.

## Final Encouragement

Sustaining growth is a never-ending adventure. By now, you have a strong foundation: self-awareness, confidence, boundary-setting, emotional resilience, financial wisdom, a sense of your values, and more. Each aspect we have discussed fits together like pieces of a puzzle, forming a more complete version of you.

No book or single resource can predict exactly what future trials or joys you will experience. But the mindset, habits, and strategies you have built will help you keep evolving with each new chapter in your life. The key is to remain curious, flexible, and kind to yourself along the way. Whether you are celebrating a triumph or stumbling through a tough season, remember that growth continues as long as you keep showing up.

# Conclusion

You have reached the end of **Women Self Improvement Book: A Woman's Guide to Personal Growth**, but your personal development story does not end here. Now is the time to apply what you have learned:

1. Keep focusing on who you are—your core values, strengths, and dreams.
2. Maintain healthy relationships and boundaries, protecting your energy so you can show up fully in the world.
3. Embrace creativity and positive thinking, staying resilient even when life becomes complicated.
4. Take charge of your finances responsibly, ensuring you have the freedom to pursue what matters to you.
5. Remember that emotional resilience helps you adapt to changes and bounce back from hardships.
6. Finally, keep growing, learning, and giving back. Use your voice and leadership qualities to influence those around you in a loving, authentic way.

Your journey is uniquely yours, filled with potential and purpose. May the lessons and insights here guide you toward a life of continued expansion, fulfillment, and joy. Whenever you feel lost, flip back to the chapters that resonate most with what you are experiencing. Let them remind you of the strong, capable woman you are—and always have been. Good luck on your path, and never stop reaching for your own definition of growth and happiness.

# Epilogue: Living Your Growth Journey

**You Are Your Greatest Ally**
Through all the chapters—exploring self-discovery, self-esteem, boundaries, communication, creativity, financial empowerment, emotional resilience, and beyond—you have seen that your most powerful partner in growth is you. The relationship you build with yourself lays the groundwork for everything else: your readiness to learn, your willingness to adapt, your capacity to love and be loved, and your drive to thrive.

Keep trusting that you are capable of ongoing transformation. Stay curious about your own thoughts and actions. Challenge yourself when you sense self-doubt creeping in. Offer yourself kind words on difficult days. By forming a supportive bond with who you are at every stage, you become a steady foundation upon which new dreams can be built.

---

**Balancing Confidence and Humility**
You have gained tools to boost confidence, but true self-assurance does not require ignoring your flaws or refusing to learn from others. Instead, it embraces a balance: you can stand tall in what you have to offer while remaining open to insights, corrections, and fresh perspectives. Confidence makes you courageous enough to try, while humility encourages you to keep growing.

Cultivating this balance will help you avoid extremes. Too little confidence can hold you back from pursuing worthy goals; too much pride can blind you to helpful feedback and new possibilities. Aim for a middle ground where you value what you bring to the table, yet also welcome advice and lessons from people whose paths or experiences differ from your own.

---

**Sustaining Healthy Habits**
The chapters touched on self-care, physical health, emotional well-being, and financial responsibility. You have learned that small actions add up—taking a short walk, saving a bit from each paycheck, enjoying a quiet moment before bed, or practicing gentle self-reflection. None of these habits need to be

overwhelming on their own. But together, they create a lifestyle where you consistently nurture your body, mind, and spirit.

If a habit slips, do not label it as total failure. Real life ebbs and flows. Instead, view each day as a chance to realign with what matters. Just like a traveler who can return to the right path after a detour, you can re-center on habits that uplift you, no matter how hectic life becomes.

---

**Relationships as a Source of Light and Lessons**

Your closest connections—family, friends, partners—reflect your capacity to give and receive support. While you cannot control every dynamic, you can decide how you respond, how you communicate, and how you set boundaries. Remember that relationships evolve over time: old friendships may fade, and new bonds may blossom. Each phase teaches you more about yourself—your desires, your tolerance, your capacity for empathy, and your willingness to stand up for your needs.

Celebrate the individuals who cheer you on and help you see your worth. Offer gratitude for those who challenge you to grow or teach you new perspectives. Even conflicts can hold a mirror up to your own behavior, revealing areas where you can become more patient, more assertive, or more loving. Let every relationship you invest in be a step toward mutual respect, shared growth, and deeper connection.

---

**Embracing the Next Chapter**

Throughout this book, you have:

- Learned to identify and honor your personal values.
- Practiced voicing your needs confidently and setting healthy boundaries.
- Strengthened your emotional and mental resilience.
- Fostered a more positive, growth-focused mindset.
- Gained practical tips to manage finances, stress, and everyday responsibilities.

Now, the next chapter of your life awaits—one that only you can write. It may involve chasing bigger dreams, learning new skills, traveling, making career moves, or pursuing deeper self-reflection. It may mean building a family or focusing on artistic expression. Whatever it is, remember that your growth does not have to match anyone else's timeline or style. You have the right to shape a path that aligns with your deepest truths.

---

**Leaving Room for Joy and Spontaneity**
With all the techniques and strategies in mind, also give yourself permission to embrace moments of unplanned joy. Personal development does not have to be a constant checklist of goals. Spontaneous fun, laughter, and creative play keep your spirit refreshed. A light heart often leads to surprising bursts of insight. Sometimes the best breakthroughs happen while you are simply enjoying life rather than trying to "fix" every aspect of yourself.

---

**Continuing Your Legacy**
As you grow, you also influence others—whether you realize it or not. Friends might notice you handling challenges with calmer composure. Younger relatives may admire your willingness to try new things or take calculated risks. Colleagues could benefit from your thoughtful listening and constructive feedback. In quiet or overt ways, you pass on the seeds of self-improvement, inspiring others to reflect on their own possibilities.

If the desire arises, formalize this positive influence by mentoring, volunteering, or sharing your experiences in a supportive community. This does not require grand gestures—a single, sincere conversation can spark an important change in someone else's journey. By paying your lessons forward, you solidify what you have learned, multiply the impact of your personal work, and help shape a kinder, more empowered society.

---

# Final Thoughts

Even the most confident, well-prepared individuals face setbacks and moments of doubt. But your resilience is now woven into every part of you, ready to cushion any falls and guide you back to your core. You have the capacity to pivot and grow through life's changes, big or small, with grace and perseverance.

You are a dynamic, evolving person—made of experiences, dreams, and undeniable strength. Keep asking questions, keep seeking truth, and keep nurturing who you are at the deepest levels. Growth is not about reaching a final state; it is about living fully, learning continuously, and bringing every part of yourself into alignment with what truly matters.

Thank you for dedicating this time to your personal development. As you step forward, may you carry curiosity, courage, and compassion for yourself and others. Your story keeps unfolding, and you hold the pen. Write it with heart, hope, and unwavering belief in your ability to shape a brighter, more authentic future—both for yourself and for those lucky enough to cross your path.

www.ingramcontent.com/pod-product-compliance
Lightning Source LLC
LaVergne TN
LVHW012109070526
838202LV00056B/5678